ME FIRST

A Guide to Honoring Your Truth,
Uncovering Your Power,
and Cultivating More Joy!

Enjoy!! :)

Copyright @ 2022 Julie Cass
Me First: A Guide to Honoring Your Truth, Uncovering Your Power, and Cultivating More Joy!
YGTMedia Co. Trade Paperback Edition.
ISBN trade paperback: 978-1-989716-66-3
eBook: 978-1-989716-67-0

All Rights Reserved. No part of this book can be scanned, distributed, or copied without permission. This book or any portion thereof may not be reproduced or used in any manner whatsoever without the express written permission of the publisher at publishing@ygtmedia.co—except for the use of brief quotations in a book review.

The author has made every effort to ensure the accuracy of the information within this book was correct at time of publication. The author does not assume and hereby disclaims any liability to any party for any loss, damage, or disruption caused by errors or omissions, whether such errors or omissions result from accident, negligence, or any other cause.

This book is designed to provide information and motivation to our readers. It is sold with the understanding that the publisher is not engaged to render any type of psychological, legal, or any other kind of professional advice. The content is the sole expression and opinion of its author, and not necessarily that of the publisher. No warranties or guarantees are expressed or implied by the publisher's choice to include any of the content in this book. Neither the publisher nor the author shall be liable for any physical, psychological, emotional, financial, or commercial damages, including, but not limited to, special, incidental, consequential or other damages. Our views and rights are the same: You are responsible for your own choices, actions, and results.

Published in Canada, for Global Distribution by YGTMedia Co.

www.ygtmedia.co/publishing

To order additional copies of this book: publishing@ygtmedia.co

Developmental editing by Tania Jane Moraes-Vaz
Edited by Christine Stock
Book design by Doris Chung
Cover design by Michelle Fairbanks
ePub edition by Ellie Silpa
Author Photo by Stacey Tarrant

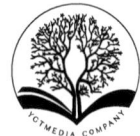

TORONTO

ME FIRST

A Guide to Honoring Your Truth,
Uncovering Your Power,
and Cultivating More Joy!

JULIE CASS

This journey of life is so much sweeter with people you love. My family and friends who have supported me and believed in me along the way, I thank you. I needed the wind in my wings to help when I had doubt.

My husband and life partner, Rob. Thank you for always believing in me and supporting me on my journey and for loving me unconditionally through the ups and downs. To my beautiful, blended family of children—Izzy, Noah, Jamison, Taylor, and Kourtney—life is sweeter and richer with you all in it. You are my biggest blessings and have taught me much. Love you always.

CONTENTS

Introduction		1
Section 1	Let's Put YOU First!	
	The Great Pause—A Quest to Finding Our Way Back to Soul	11
Chapter 1	What Is the Point, Mom?	15
Chapter 2	Why Are We So Unhappy?	23
Chapter 3	Why Does This Keep Happening to Me?	35
Chapter 4	Conscious Forgiveness	47
Chapter 5	Judgment, What Gives? Shift from Judgment to Love	63
Chapter 6	Healing Our Inner Critic and Loving Our Perfectly Imperfect Selves	73
Chapter 7	Who Says You Can't Have It All?	83
Chapter 8	I Have Never Felt Safe to Relax	93
Chapter 9	Working from a Place of Inspiration versus Hustle	107
Chapter 10	Who Am I to Do This, Desire This, Be This?	123
Chapter 11	Our Differences Are What Make Us Human	131
Chapter 12	Curiosity Allows Expansion	143
Chapter 13	Power of Choice	153

Chapter 14	Trusting Self Is the Only Way	163
Chapter 15	You Living Your Truth Is a Gift	169
Chapter 16	Some Days You Need Potato Salad and Chocolate	187

Section 2	Let's Discover Your Power + Simplify Your Life + Birth Your Desire: The Road Map to Fulfilling Your Heartfelt Desires	
	The Road Map	195
Chapter 17	Uncover Your Power—Taking 100 Percent Responsibility	201
Chapter 18	Fertilizing Your Desires	215
Chapter 19	The Power of Your Mind	231
Chapter 20	Your Why	241
Chapter 21	What Gets in Your Way	247
Chapter 22	Mastering the Creation Cycle	265
Chapter 23	Putting "Me" into Loving Action	271
Conclusion	What Is the Point? Coming Full Circle	279
	Acknowledgments	285
	Resources and Works Cited	289

INTRODUCTION

I know, you're probably wondering, *How on earth can you name a book* Me First *without sounding pigheaded, stuck-up, and full of yourself?*

This thought ran through my head more than once as I wrote this book. But the truth is, the whole meaning of this book is to understand why we have to put ourselves first and fall deeply and completely in love with ourselves in order to live a life that not only looks good on the outside but also feels good on the inside.

Me First talks about loving yourself through it all. The kind of love that is deep, raw, uninhibited. The kind of love that looks at the internal dialogue we have with ourselves in each moment and the messages we tell ourselves every single day that ultimately shape our beliefs and thus ultimately shape our experiences.

It means digging deep at the core and understanding more about *who you are being*, 24 hours a day, 365 days a year.

You're the only person who knows exactly how and why you behave/act/think/speak the way you do—to yourself and others. You are the only person who is intimately with yourself in each moment.

If we don't love who we are and how we show up during every minute of the day, how can we show up as our highest and best self in the world? How can we attract the love that we really want until we love ourselves deeply?

It's not possible. Or, what happens is this: *How* you show up and the kinds of circumstances, people, and opportunities that show up for you in your life are an exact replica of your thoughts, your mindset, your perspective on life. It's a glass half full or half empty kinda situation.

So, *Me First* is about getting really cozy and comfortable with being who you are—putting yourself first in every way. And if it makes you uncomfortable to read the title, that's a good thing. It was for me. I had to stretch my own beliefs and realize that until I became comfortable with this notion of really choosing myself first, I couldn't be truly happy. Until I became comfortable with the notion that choosing me first doesn't make me selfish and that it's quite the contrary, I couldn't truly be happy. Putting myself first is actually the most unselfish thing I can do, and the only thing I should be doing is really understanding who I am at my core—us. Me, I, the one.

What I realized, and believe, is this: Every single time I feel triggered by events, people, actions, or what others do, it means there is a need for deeper healing within myself. So, *Me First* is a journey into the depths of your own healing. It's a deep ride that plummets you off the mountain, causing you to dive into the depths of your soul to figure out *how, when, where,* and *what* you need to do to live your fullest, richest, deepest, most loving life.

Me First is a reclamation and rediscovery of how intricate your mind, body, and soul are. It's an uncovering of all the layers and nuances you hold within your body—every cell, every word, every thought, every action. It is a rediscovery of your power and potential and how you are truly capable of creating anything you desire. It is the song that will guide you home to yourself as you explore all the crevices, cracks, and depths that make you who you are.

Me First is a declaration that you are worth exploring; you are worth getting intimately involved with. You are worth falling in love with, more and more each day. Yes, that maddening, deep, intense kind of love. The type that has your back, no matter what. The gentle, soothing, powerful love that also knows how to hold space for all the wounds and scars that will come up for air and healing. You are worthy of discovering the powerhouse that you have within you.

The relationship you have with yourself is ultimately the biggest thing that will dictate *what* you get to experience in your outer world and *how* you navigate it. Digging deep and choosing to understand who you are and what you desire and what your path is and how you can grow every day will not only help you find inner peace but will also BE PEACE. It will help you not only find love but also BE LOVE. It will help you not only reach for joy but also emanate JOY on this path of life.

The purpose of our life as we know it is to evolve, ascend, or master it.

But I ask you this . . .

Do you believe you are worthy of loving yourself enough to live your best life?

My hope is for you to take this journey with me and discover how powerful you are. This is your invitation, your initiation to shift from being the victim in your life to being the hero or heroine by taking full responsibility for your thoughts, your actions, and your behaviors. When you live from a "me first" mentality, you take full responsibility for your own life. I believe we try too hard to be responsible for other people's lives, and it is not only a thankless job, but it is also an impossible one, with heartache as its only reward. I learned the hard way that it is not our job to be responsible for anyone else (other than young children who rely on us). In this context, when you take full responsibility for your life, you raise your energetic vibration. When you do this, everyone around you benefits, and they ultimately shift. As a mom, I learned that being a martyr was the worst thing I could do for my children. I was angry, resentful, and ultimately, not joyful. Instead, when I prioritized my well-being *and* my evolution, my kids benefited in such an impactful way, far more than when I was playing the role of martyr or savior. They did not deserve that version of me. The only commonality? I was, and still am, the only one who can make that choice for myself.

Today, if I find myself going to a place of anger (which definitely happens), the first thing I ask myself is: *What is it within me that needs to be healed?* There are many, many days when I find myself still wanting to blame others for my pain, but I know that staying in that spiral isn't beneficial for me or anyone else. So I remind myself that the only way out of any lower emotion is to feel it in order to heal it and to take responsibility for my own emotions. To look within first. To look at me first.

For me, this is the most empowering way to live. It allows me to shift into alignment faster rather than lingering in misery for way too long, which is something I used to do (and believe many of us do). It is my desire and intention for you to use this book as a guide, a stepping-stone to putting yourself first.

So, get cozy, grab a cup of tea, and let's take this journey to what it means to be 100 percent responsible, which will ultimately allow you to tap into more joy!

HOW TO READ THIS BOOK

There is no right or wrong way to read this book. All I ask of you as you read it is to give yourself grace, get comfortable and cozy, and read a page or two, or more.

Do what feels best for you. Stay open to what surfaces. If you feel like you need a pause, allow yourself that.

There is no chronological order to this book. Feel free to open to a chapter in the beginning, middle, or end.

In the first half of the book, we explore concepts of consciousness, beliefs, mindset, choice, curiosity, and navigating emotions, to name a few. Each of these have a ME FIRST manifesto at the end—you can screenshot it, write it in your journal, and/or share it with a friend or loved one who needs it. There are exercises and meditations (written and audio) woven throughout that you can immerse yourself in. See the Resources section for a playlist you can listen to while reading this book.

The second half of the book contains my core teachings and visual aids to help guide you along the way. I recommend choosing one chapter a week so you can ground and integrate each of these teachings and experience the micro and macro shifts in your life.

It is my sincere desire for this book to be an immersive, expansive, and life-changing experience for you.

I'd love to hear from you as you take this journey to finally living a life that is centered on the principles of *Me First*. Feel free to reach out to me on Instagram @thepositivechangegroup, www.thepositivechangegroup.com, or julie@thepositivechange.com

With love,

Julie Cass

SECTION 1

LET'S PUT YOU FIRST!

THE GREAT PAUSE–A QUEST TO FINDING OUR WAY BACK TO SOUL

The world has changed rapidly in the last two years since 2020—in some ways, more so than it ever has in our lifetime. What once felt safe—simple human interaction—is now viewed as dangerous, harmful, contagious. We have been asked throughout the last two years to go against our natural instincts as humans and distance from one another. We have been asked to spend time away from our loved ones because it is considered dangerous to see each other.

    I like to call the last two years The Great Pause. Others call them The Great Reset. Perhaps they are a pause *and* a reset. The typical routine "busyness" of our calendars has been cleared, while also feeling full. Many people now face a void for the first time in their lives—a pause and a surplus of time to just be! Yes, some people now work from home (for all the jobs that allowed for it), but others lost their jobs or chose to start a new venture, something they may never had pursued had it not been for The Great Pause. And for others, this pause made them feel uncomfortable because their usual distractions in life were eliminated.

When we are faced with a trauma or situations that bring up fear because they are out of our control, we are compressed to a point where it is uncomfortable. It is like squeezing a stress ball that deflates and compacts when tension is applied to it. But the beauty is that compression and tension then lead to expansion or "growth."

When we are in darkness, we can see the light, even if it is a glimmer.

I believe this to be true for what we are currently experiencing. It is a compression, a time of tension, a time when we are each called to lead—ourselves and others—to be the light, a time when we are asked to explore our truth and to feel every single emotion. It is also a time that has created a space to look deeper within, a space to get in touch with ourselves to examine our values, re-prioritize what matters, and become intentional and aware of how we choose to spend our time and energy. It has created an unearthing of issues that we might have buried for so long because we were once too "busy" with life and too distracted by our own deeper truths and emotions.

When I look back on my life, my biggest growth opportunities have always resulted from some of my hardest, lowest moments. I bet the same is true for you. We might not see it in the moment, but in hindsight, we realize that there is always a blessing and a lesson built into every experience.

I believe we are creating a necessary shift in consciousness on the planet. We are all part of this shift. If you are brave enough to not run away from the problems at hand and instead invite your curiosity about what this time in history can mean for you, then ask yourself these questions:

How can you live a life with a deeper connection to self?

What can you say no to that drains your energy, and what can you choose more of that raises your vibration?

How can you move more in alignment with who you are, every single day?

Never has there been a more important time to live your truth, speak your truth, empower yourself to your greatest potential, raise your energy vibration, and find your liberation. I believe this space in time has been created for all of us to do exactly that—to become more discerning of what we want, to step into our worthiness and be able to receive more, and ultimately, to cultivate a deeper love and connection to self.

I hope you enjoy this journey with me in *Me First*. I hope you lean into your courage, into the discomfort of unpacking what has held you back for so many years from living a truth-filled life. I invite you to assess everything that has been contributing to you living out of your powerful alignment. This journey is about choosing to get to know yourself, love yourself, and live in your power. That is the biggest impact you can have on this world.

Enjoy!

CHAPTER 1

WHAT IS THE POINT, MOM?

It's morning, and I was getting ready to head to my office. I was brushing my teeth in the bathroom when my daughter walked in. I could tell she felt like talking because she was lingering around. When your teenage daughter feels like talking to you, as a parent, you linger too, because it is a rare moment.

"How's it going, Izz?" I asked.

"Well, okay, Mom, I guess. I just, I don't know, I am wondering something."

"Cool. Like what?" I asked, trying to play it casual so she would open up and keep talking.

She blurted out, "Like what is the whole point to this anyway? What is the purpose of waking up, going to school, then repeating it the next day? Nothing really changes, and it just seems a bit useless. I mean, what is really the point to all this?"

Well, *that's* a loaded question, and it came before I'd even had my morning coffee. But it's a good question nonetheless, one that I know I have asked myself several times as I am sure you have too. Now, at the time that my daughter asked this question, we happened to have been in the COVID-19 pandemic for more than a year, and it did feel like Groundhog Day, over and over again. I'm sure this was partly why she was asking this simple yet profound question: "What is the point, Mom?"

And I would guess that this time in history has made many people get curious as to what the point is and what really matters.

"Hmm," I responded, taking my time to answer. "Well, I believe the whole point to this life is to experience as much joy and happiness as you possibly can. To linger in happiness, to do things that make you happy, to be with people that make you happy, and to make choices that can bring you more happiness. And most importantly, it is to love who you are so you can really feel that happiness. Otherwise, what is the point?"

She looked at me with wide eyes, and I could sense her head spinning inside.

"That's why, Izzy, if something makes you happy, then you should do it. And if you can't seem to figure out what that is, then get curious and spend time figuring that out. The answer will come. And if it doesn't bring you joy, then stop doing it. Whatever that is, except for school, of course." I then give her a wink and ask for a hug. "Hugging you brings me joy," I said as I squeezed her tight.

She grunted, as teenagers do, then walked off. Well, maybe that would give her something to ponder for the day.

I wish that I had, at a younger age, gotten curious enough to ask that question. I mean, I guess my parents gave me that same message, but I never really felt safe to choose my unique path. I felt that my happiness was dependent on theirs. My happiness had to fit within the family expectations, and it needed to make them happy as well. The happiness I believed in as a kid had its limitations and boundaries. It was not free flowing, and at times, I felt shame for wanting certain things as they were not "appropriate." I realized over the years that this flawed concept of limiting my happiness to suit others started to shape my life and my choices.

 Are you truly living every day with a consciousness around cultivating more happiness?

No really, take a moment and think about it.

I deeply believe if more people lived this way, the world would be a better place. I believe we would have less judgment and resentment toward others. I believe there would be less anger and hatred. You see, it is impossible to be happy and bitter at the same time. It is impossible to feel true love for ourselves and then hatred for others. The two emotions cannot coexist.

My aha: We are all connected.

What does that mean?

This awareness took me years to understand and actually conceptualize.

 Think about this: If we are truly all connected, then if I hate another, I hate myself. If I am angry at someone else, then I am angry at myself. If I judge another, I judge myself. If I hold resentment toward someone else, then I am resentful toward myself.

The deeper you fall in love with yourself, the less you hate others because it is impossible. The more you forgive yourself, the greater your capacity is to forgive others.

If such is the case, would it not make sense that we cultivate this relationship with self first? That we make ourselves a priority? That "me first" is actually our path to liberation, freedom, and love?

I know you're nodding your head as you read these words.

Here's the hard part: The truth is that for many of us, the hardest part is releasing the lifelong conditioning or coding that has impregnated our minds. We were not taught to make happiness a priority. Instead, we were asked to lean into the hustle, struggle, suffering, lack, limitations, and fear. Instead of choosing our needs, wants, and desires first, we were told that we must think of others first or we would be "selfish." And if this strikes a chord with you right now, lean into that. There is something there that is coming up for healing. When someone calls you selfish, it feels awful. We feel shame in our bodies. We think thoughts like *How could I be so selfish?* and *How can they think I am selfish?* So, we do things we really don't want to do so others will never judge us in that way again and because we want to avoid that feeling at all costs. This creates a cycle of neglecting our own wants, desires, and needs to the point where we forget how to choose self-love because it is such a foreign concept. It feels so unfamiliar and awkward. Anger, resentment, and bitterness feel more familiar to us, so we perpetuate this pattern and create a vicious cycle. The further we stray from our truth, the deeper the anger and hatred becomes.

The only path to freedom and living a liberated life that feels good inside out is to unapologetically choose yourself first. Love yourself the deepest. By doing so, you cannot hate, judge, or condemn because you won't like how that feels in your own body. When you love yourself deeper, the world gets the best of you, and you create ripples of positivity and light that touch so many people.

In this book, we explore and uncover simple techniques and processes for how you can choose yourself first, love yourself deeper, cultivate more happiness, attract your most heartfelt desire with ease, and be in complete alignment with your path and destiny, where joy is the only option.

"Me first" is not only about choosing to love yourself unconditionally, it is also about taking full responsibility for your life, your actions, your words, and your behaviors.

When we don't have a "me first" attitude, we look to blame others or the world for our unhappiness. We lean into anger or hate so easily because we see ugliness in others. What we fail to realize is that when we focus on the negativity, ugliness, and annoyances in others, it is a mere reflection of what we see in ourselves.

Therefore, the concept of "me first" means looking within *first* whenever we feel activated, triggered, hurt, or sad.

"Me first" means asking yourself the question: What is this opportunity trying to teach me, as I feel triggered by ____.

"Me first" means we recognize that there is always something in us that needs healing or loving if we feel anger and hate toward someone else.

"Me first" is the most unselfish way to live because we don't choose to jump to blame or judgment, even though it can feel so much easier to do so.

"Me first" means loving yourself truly, deeply, and with devotion so that you can love others more. It means connecting with yourself so you can connect with others. It means filling your own cup first so your resources aren't depleted and you can pour freely, out of love and service—not obligation—into others.

ME FIRST **means I love myself, and I love others too, but not at the expense of myself.**
ME FIRST **means choosing myself over and over again, so that I can lead myself and others in the most aligned manner.**
ME FIRST **means living in alignment with my truth while honoring and respecting others' truths.**

CHAPTER 2

WHY ARE WE SO UNHAPPY?

Why are we unhappy as a collective?

Why is there so much pain and suffering?

How can there be a God when there is pain?

If God or some higher power exists, the world wouldn't be in a state of chaos and disaster right now . . .

Have you ever thought these things?

Have you ever asked yourself these questions?

I know I did.

Why do bad things happen to good people? Is there someone in the clouds who keeps score of whether you were naughty or nice, good or bad, enough or not enough? Is there someone up there who determines how well you did or didn't do today and decides what your reward will be? Is there someone out there who keeps tabs on your suffering, your happiness, your pain and sorrow and then randomly decides that *you've suffered enough, now you get to live and be at peace*? Or *you are a good person so you will not suffer*? That doesn't seem to be the case.

And so many of us put this faith in a "god" to save us and even the score. We assign our power to some celestial being who is tracking the good and bad and deciding who gets what. Here's the problem with this way of thinking: When things go our way, our faith deepens, and everything is wonderful in our world. But when things don't go our way, we lose faith, we get angry, and we become desperate to understand why things don't work out in our favor or why we don't get what we asked or "prayed" for.

I believe in being able to surrender wholly and trusting the process while still taking responsibility for my life and how I desire to feel. I am all for prayers and trusting in a higher power (God, Universe, Source, whatever you believe in), but I don't believe in handing over our personal power and God/Source-given ability to do something about a situation or circumstance outside of ourselves to something outside of ourselves.

Looking outside of ourselves for the answers creates a huge sense of unhappiness within the collective. We believe that we have to simply react to the cards that have been dealt to us. We believe that none of it is in our control. We believe that someone else or something else can make us happy. We might even believe that someone else is responsible for our happiness. But then we become bitter and resentful at the world because it is not fair. If you believe in God, or some higher power, you might start to question your faith. We become the victim and the martyr of our life. We feel powerless and at the mercy of others.

Yuck! This is no way to live. And yet many of us are in this stuck place. I know I was for a very long time. I lived from a place of fear and worry, and I always wondered when the other shoe would drop. In fact, whenever I felt happy, part of me felt like I would be cursed and damned for feeling too good, so I would go back to worrying. Worry and fear actually felt more comfortable for me than happiness. It felt safer. It felt more familiar. It's the energetic vibration that felt comfortable within my body—known and familiar.

But this is insane when you think about it. We can literally train ourselves to be more comfortable with fear than happiness. More familiar with anger than love. And so, we hold ourselves back and stop ourselves from living in our freedom and happiness. But the key is *we* do this to ourselves when, in fact, we are responsible for this life of ours. When we are in fear and anger, we perpetuate more things to be fearful and angry about. We literally attract those emotions into our life.

My life changed when I hit my rock bottom. I knew that I hated the life I was living *and* that I also had to take full responsibility for it. I cracked the code to life when I realized I couldn't blame anyone or anything for my own unhappiness. I was fully responsible. Not a celestial being in the sky, not my ex-husband or my parents. Nope, it was me.

I had to look in the mirror and ask myself a freakin' scary question: *What are you going to do about it, Julie?*

When we take full responsibility for our misery, we can take full responsibility for our happiness and realize that *we* hold the key to both outcomes. I quickly learned that this is the most empowering and fulfilling way to live and that we are such powerful beings who create our reality every day. Every moment is a creation. Every thought is a seed of creation in your garden. Every action is a step closer to an outcome that you are creating.

LOOKING AT OUR SHIT TO SHIFT

In my life, the times I have felt most miserable is when I felt completely out of control. I felt powerless because I believed I was at the mercy of others—their viewpoints, opinions, judgments, and rules.

I remember feeling such a heaviness in my chest that, at times, I literally thought it would burst wide open. I so badly desired the recognition I felt I deserved. I felt like I was starving for it. And when I didn't get it based on my expectations, it felt awful. I felt heavy and defeated by life. I felt like it didn't matter what I did, it would never be enough. My personal interpretation was: "I will never be enough."

I was miserable. This belief that I adopted was making me miserable.

My self-talk: *Breathe, wipe the tears away, Julie. Take a deep breath and try to pull yourself out of this drama and see it for what it really is.*

I was miserable because I gave away all my power. I thought I needed validation from someone else to feel my own sense of worth because mine was not strong enough for me. I expected love and nourishment from others when I didn't and couldn't give that to myself, and I was disappointed.

But ultimately, it was a gift.

It was a gift because it showed me that I kept giving away my power and expecting an outcome based on someone else's actions. It showed me that the only one in charge of me, is me.

I can only control and govern myself. I can love myself deeper, then increase my capacity to love others and not be wounded so incredibly by others' actions or lack of actions.

Being anchored in my truth of who I am as a human being is the gift. I take back my power and no longer allow anyone else's comments, thoughts, or negativity to land on me or to take up the energetic space they used to. Rather than seething with anger, I can now be compassionate toward others and myself. I can show love and kindness toward others and myself. I am not dependent on outside validation.

Now, don't get me wrong; I am human, of course, and so are you. I love being validated, and I love getting recognition from others, but I have learned to embrace it when it happens instead of solely relying on it to get me through my day-to-day. The fundamental difference is not depending on it for your sense of worth and happiness. And the only way that happens is when you are in your center, when you are in love with who you are—flaws and all! Because when you are rooted in your core values, in your center, when you are living your truth and loving yourself, only the highest and best parts of you come to life. Literally the best part of you comes to life, living your life. And when you resonate and reverberate at that energy and frequency, not only do others' opinions *not* throw you off anymore, but your energy also becomes so powerful that it shifts others around you. We are energy. Everything around us is made of energetic vibrations. So, the higher your frequency, the more likely that people around you will feel it and inevitably shift—they will rise to meet you where you're at, or they'll show themselves out of your life.

I believe that we are often miserable and unhappy with ourselves, our life, and everything else that goes with it because we have not taken full responsibility for our life. We have not yet fallen in love with ourselves, and we look for outside validation to find the love we are starved for receiving. We are at the whim of how others treat us or what they say to us.

I'm looking at the trees outside my office right now, and they are blowing to the south instead of the west because there is a northerly wind. They are responding and reacting to the direction of the wind. However, their roots are planted solid in the ground. They do not move. The tree knows its true self. Grounded and solid in Mother Nature and connected to Source. The more mature the tree, the more mature the roots.

We are like trees. The more we live and the more we experience, the bigger our roots and the more solid our foundation. The more inner work we do, the more we return home to our roots, our true self, our connection to that which is greater. We may blow in the wind, sometimes even bend or break and adapt accordingly to the climate and conditions as they change around us, but we always know who we are.

When I allow my heart to break as a result of another's action, I break a piece of me, like a branch falling off. I have become weak rather than just letting the wind or comments blow past me. Maybe I would have swayed a bit with the wind or comment, but all I had to do was go back to my roots, my truth of who I am, and not let it break me. It only has the power to break me or make me miserable if I let it.

If we take these opportunities of heartbreak and use them for transformation, we can grow stronger by using the experience and lesson within it to heal a part of ourselves that probably needs it. We strengthen our emotional center. Not only do we heal, but we become more capable and stronger than before. "Me first" means digging deeper into your truth, being your biggest cheerleader, and carving your own path that you are destined to have.

When you find yourself not living your unique path and instead doing things based on expectations or obligations, you will never find your inner peace. It is impossible because you are uniquely you. Someone else's path could never possibly be your own. Their opinion will not make you more whole. I have tried that before, and it didn't work. The only thing that is constant and certain is knowing your roots, your truth. And when a harsh/insensitive/

thoughtless comment comes your way, rather than it breaking your heart, just let your leaves rustle in the wind and quietly thank them for the opportunity to heal another piece of you inside that needs love.

Every single thing that occurs in our life is for our growth or healing. We are complex beings, yes. Like an onion, we, too, have many layers to our humanness, our way of being, our emotions. The more layers we are willing to peel back or have the courage to look at, the sweeter the center of this life gets. The juicier self and parts of life get to play out. The richest and most potent self gets to shine. And that, my friend, is happiness. That is truth—our roots and who we truly are.

Perhaps you're reading and wondering, *Hmm, Julie, why are so many people miserable?* I personally believe it is a measure of their willingness to look at their own shit. Are they willing to dig deep and peel back the layers of the onion to get to the sweet, juicy center? Or do they shy away at the first sign of discomfort? You are the only one who can decide *when* you do this for yourself. The minute you blame someone else means you are not looking at your own layer—you are projecting on others instead.

Does it feel like some of us have more shit than others?

Yes, of course it does. But that does not mean you are faulty or less worthy. It is exactly what you have needed to happen for your growth. When I look back on my life, the hardest, darkest days have spawned the most light in my life because they gave me the seeds of inspiration to grow, to uncover all that needed to be uncovered, and to align myself to my truth and discover what exactly my truth was anyway. *Who am I? What am I here to do?*

I listen to that inner calling and voice more frequently now to guide me, to lead me, to be my inspiration. And I believe when we do that, we don't need to have the deepest valleys of despair, because we are living from a place of inspiration and love rather than hate, anger, and memories. When we live from a place of love versus fear, we are led to love, we feel more love, and we feel safe because we *are* safe and nurtured.

Years ago, my yoga master told me, "We live in a mirroring universe." I may not have fully comprehended the meaning at the time, but I realize in hindsight just how true it is. When I lived my life from a place of fear, I had more fear in my life. I had more anxiety. When I live from a place of trust and love, things just are more trusting and loving. I don't attract the things I fear. We are like magnets.

What are you attracted to in your life?

If you are filled with fear, you attract more things to fear. If you are constantly sucked into the drama and gossip around you, it is natural that you will attract more things to be dramatic about. But the beauty is that when you're done with it, you literally can decide to be done with it. You make different choices, you might hang with different friends, you might attract a new soul community of people that is more in alignment with you. But here is the key. **You get to decide, always!**

So, is it worth looking at your SHIT?

You decide.

If you think it is, then let's do a little exercise:

Write down three things you would like to shift in your life that you are not happy with:

1.
2.
3.

Now, review the list and assess how many things on it are about you or someone else. If it had anything to do with someone else, then rewrite it—this time with you taking full responsibility. What is it within you that needs to shift?

1.
2.
3.

Great! Now you have the power to shift. But it has to be in full responsibility. Remember, you cannot shift anyone else or do the work for anyone else. You can only do it for yourself. Now ask yourself:

What are these three things here to teach me? What can they do for me? What is the blessing from these things?

1.
2.
3.

There is always a blessing under the shit. Always. If you are having a hard time finding it, that is okay. It just might take some more time. But a good way to get there is to really examine the trigger. As humans, our triggers inevitably boil down to our basic needs not being met: love, safety, or belonging. Try to categorize it into one of those triggers that needs to be healed.

ME FIRST **is an understanding of the soul contract—it has been preparing for both the darkness and the lightness of life for lifetimes, so you can finally put yourself first and discover who you are.**

CHAPTER 3

WHY DOES THIS KEEP HAPPENING TO ME?

Ever wonder why something keeps happening over and over again? It keeps recurring like a time loop that you feel trapped in. Or perhaps you keep running into the same type of circumstance or scenario, but with different people?

I have the answer for you . . . are you ready?

It's because you have yet to learn the lesson. YOU are the commonality between all these situations—perhaps it's your behavior, your thoughts, or perhaps it's this . . .

You are still taking the pieces or fragmented parts of you with yourself into every experience you walk into and choose.

For instance, one morning I went for a beautiful bike ride with a friend of mine who I know is struggling. He asked if he could have my perspective on things. He felt angry and resentful that his marriage fell apart and his wife left.

"What is going on for you now?" I asked.

"Well, you know the saying, 'three strikes and you are out'? This is my third relationship, and I don't want this to happen to me again. So, I don't want to risk it again by putting myself out there."

"Hmm . . ." I said. "Yup, I can understand how that can be scary. So, do you actually think three *failed* relationships is a lot? And just because a relationship doesn't last forever, is it actually a failure?"

"Well, you know what they say, if you can't make it the third time, chances are you can't make it and it will happen again."

"You're right," I said. "But the chances of you having a breakup again have nothing to do with how many *failed* relationships you have had in the past." (I say failed as a response to him, but not because I believe a relationship breaking is a failure. In fact, there are so many beautiful things that have come from his marriage: his two beautiful kids, years of friendship, years of growth and self-discovery, if you are willing to see it through that lens, but I find a lot of people don't because it is just easier to stay mad and resentful.)

"The reason it will happen again is because you believe it will. You have already decided that based on your past," I told him.

"What else am I supposed to believe, Julie? This keeps happening to me!"

It was a lovely morning. I was grateful for the time we had to talk and the fact that we were in nature because I believe nature always gives us the grounding that we need. I took a deep breath and really thought about how to answer this question. I didn't want to sound preachy or like I was lecturing him, but what I really wanted to say was this: "Get your head out of your ass, look in the mirror, and take responsibility for your life because nothing is happening **to** you. It is happening **for** you to look at yourself—to love yourself deeper and to decide that you are worthy and that you can break this pattern if you want and if you are willing to choose it." *Sigh*. I took another deep breath and looked around at the beauty as we rode our bikes.

I probed further. "What makes you think that it will happen again; what makes you believe that? And don't say it is because this is your third relationship, because most people your age have had many more than three relationships in their lifetime, so what else?"

I was trying to get to the core belief because until we get there, we make analogies and excuses in our life because it is easier. And we all do it. These excuses distract us from the truth—the truth of what we believe to be true about ourselves.

We kept pedaling. There was silence for a while and then he said, "If she doesn't feel like I am good enough, then who will? I was not enough for her, so I am not sure who I will be enough for. . . ."

And there it was: The core belief of *I am not enough*!

UNCOVERING YOUR ENOUGHNESS

Why do we allow others to dictate our sense of enoughness? Who decides whether we are good enough? If we are enough, at all? For a large part of my life, I have identified with this belief. There are still times when it trickles in and I am so aware of it that it actually pisses me off because I have worked on this limiting belief for years. This limiting belief can rear its ugly head in struggling relationships, money blocks, obstacles in building a business . . . you name it, I can bet it is there when an obstacle arises. In almost any situation where we get stuck, if we dig deep there is a voice somewhere inside that says, *Who says? Who do you think you are? Good luck, you can't.* And ultimately, *You are not good enough!*

So, I couldn't judge him for thinking this thought. We have all been plagued by it to varying degrees. But I do know there is only one way out of this spin cycle and that he will keep repeating the pattern until he awakes to the truth.

"Thanks for sharing that with me. Thank you for trusting me with your truth. Let me ask you this: Do you think you are a good person?"

"Well, yes, I do," he said with passion.

"Do you think you have a lot to offer someone in a relationship?"

"Yes, but clearly, she didn't, nor did anyone else," he said, slipping back into the martyr and victim role.

"Okay, can you list some of the things you love or like about yourself?"

"I am thoughtful, kind, and loyal. I love the outdoors and being active. I am trustworthy," he said.

"Amazing. So do you believe you have a lot to offer and would be a great catch?"

"Hmm, I can easily see how I would be but clearly it is not enough to be all of those things for someone else," he said, again believing that he's not in control of his life or anything—everything depends on how someone else treats him.

"The most important thing is that you believe them to be true. It is the only thing. And when your wife wants to break up, it becomes even more important for you to believe those things about yourself. To anchor yourself in that truth. The more you believe in yourself and your qualities, the easier it is to attract the right fit—the person who prioritizes those qualities too. But if you let your sense of self-worth be determined by others' perceptions, you will never feel whole. In fact, it will keep showing itself again and again until you start looking inward and know that it's always within you. That is what I believe. The universe mirrors what is going on inside of us."

"So you have two choices here," I said.

1. "Stay in self-pity, anger, and resentment. If you keep hating her, you keep hating yourself. You can keep blaming her for the fallout and take no responsibility on your part. Not the best path to inner peace and happiness.

OR

2. "Work on deeply knowing your self-worth, qualities, and what makes you special and believing in them and who you are—wholeheartedly. Repeat these in your mind, feel them in your heart and soul, become unshakable in your truth of who you really are. AND take responsibility for your part. Look at your part of the equation. Choose to learn from the experience. Remember, you take **you** with you everywhere you go. You can take the path to being broken on this journey or you can take the path of self-reflection and healing."

Okay, I know, I know, I might have sounded preachy after saying all of that! But he thanked me, and we made plans to see each other with our kids over the weekend. My advice or my truth did not push him away. I gave him the same advice I give myself over and over, which is to ask myself the question: *What is my part here, in this situation, in this relationship dynamic?* Blaming someone or something, living by the belief of *Why is this happening to me?* will never get you out of the spin cycle of anger, despair, and unhappiness.

Reflecting upon why something has happened *for* us is the path to growth, healing, love, and ultimate freedom from the shackles in our mind of anger and resentment.

I remember reading *The Big Leap* by Gay Hendricks a few years back. There was a part of the book when he was talking about relationships that really stuck out for me: In a relationship, you are both 100 percent responsible.

At the time I said, "How is that possible?" All my fights with my husband are about the other person taking responsibility for their actions. And then we would fight over which one of us is at fault the most. Actually, we have wasted a lot of time and energy over the years in making the other person responsible. So, the "100 percent each" made me uncomfortable. If that was the case, then I couldn't be so angry, I couldn't put my foot in the sand

and make my point or scream until I felt heard. I realized what made me uncomfortable was that this was a pattern I was used to, even if it always made me feel like shit and sometimes took me days to recover from.

In a relationship, if both you and your partner are 100 percent responsible, then instead of placing blame, start looking within—examine the role you play within your relationship, your learning, and your growth, and understand your triggers and why you have them. I truly believe a trigger is a sign that something within you needs to be healed.

OH, but that is heavy lifting. It feels uncomfortable, which is why most of us are unwilling to look at that. Anger is so much easier to feel than taking responsibility. So, we stay in the spin cycle.

Personally, I also found that in my relationships, I'd let my pride get in the way and stop me from owning my part. It felt much easier to place blame instead. Judging others was easier than claiming full responsibility for how *I* showed up in any of my relationships.

My bike ride that morning with my friend reminded me of exactly this. I can so clearly see it like a movie playing out in front of me when it is happening to someone else. I can even predict the next scene that will happen based on the beliefs the person is holding on to. If you want a different scene in the movie, you have to change the roles of your beliefs. You have to identify the core belief and then look at how to upgrade it. Then the characters get to show up in a different way; they get to demand different things out of life, all based on their beliefs and perceptions. A belief will allow you to demand more for yourself or become complacent and status quo. A belief will allow you to take charge or become a victim.

The belief of this is happening *to* me versus *for* me is a good place to start.

So, Julie, when is it time to move on from victimhood?

As soon as you can without pretending you are okay.

The key here is to not pretend. Pretending you are okay will just prolong the agony. We are human and we have emotions. We need to feel our emotions and not be afraid or ashamed of them. We also need to understand the power these emotions have on us. Anger is a very low energetic vibration. When we feel angry, we also feel and take on the frequency of anger in our bodies. If we choose to linger in this frequency, we see disharmony show up physically, not just emotionally.

As a trained practitioner in Emotional Freedom Technique (EFT), one of the core teachings is that all physical issues have an energetic block. If you study Traditional Chinese Medicine

(TCM), there is also the belief that any blocks in our meridians or energy channels have physical alignments associated with them. Yoga, which dates back thousands of years, has the chakra system whereby each chakra or main energy center within our bodies relates to different emotional frequencies. When our chakras/meridians/energy centers are blocked or stagnant, physical ailments manifest. When they aren't clear-flowing channels of high energetic vibrations such as love, joy, forgiveness, peace, etc., it can show up in our bodies.

If you're wondering what on earth I'm talking about, it's okay, I get it. I felt the same way when I first heard about it. But here's the thing: You already know what being in a low vibrational state versus a high vibrational state feels like in your body. You've felt it before. Think about it for a minute. When you are angry, you feel like shit. When you are in love, you feel ecstasy. So, how long do you want to linger and feel those lower emotions of anger and resentment or jealousy and shame or guilt?

I could see my friend suffering. He wanted to lean into his anger and blame his ex-wife for his unhappiness.

"The angrier you get with her, the more you suffer. You may think that you are punishing her by being mad at her, but you are actually just punishing yourself because staying angry is making you feel like shit." Thank goodness we were on our bikes so he didn't deck me. It might not have been what he wanted to hear, but it's the truth and the only way out. I know this from my own experience.

Allow yourself to feel sad. Don't ignore the grieving process. We need to experience the full range of our emotions instead of denying them or numbing their release.

"Yes, it does suck that your marriage ended. I wish it could be different for both of you—I wish you could have both been happy in this marriage," I said. "But that is not the case, so now what? How long do you want to stay mad? Maybe go out to the middle of a field, yell, scream, and get your rage out. Then allow yourself to have a good cathartic cry. Don't deny the emotions. Look them in the face and really feel them." I told him this because that is the first step to transitioning through to the other side.

I believe we need to affirm the emotion rather than deny it. When we can affirm it, we gain clarity and can then work on the healing journey. We can transition into higher emotions faster, in deeper alignment with ourselves.

Once you look your anger in the eye, instead of accepting it as your reality, ask yourself, "How do I pick up the pieces and not only get my life back but also make it better than what it used to be? How do I look at this and actually see the blessings that are here for me, because this is not happening *to* me but *for* me?"

ME FIRST **means taking responsibility and owning my part so I can shift into perspective way faster and ultimately, my experience.**

CHAPTER 4

CONSCIOUS FORGIVENESS

Do you find that you forgive yourself and others easily? Or do you tend to hang onto misgivings and grudges? Whichever end of the spectrum you resonate with, give yourself grace. You are human. Forgiveness doesn't always come easily to us because we typically remember every single word, thought, and action. But here is my unpopular opinion: Forgiveness is freedom. It is a tool that we all have access to and yet many of us don't use it. Instead, we hang on to anger and resentment of others because we feel that to forgive would mean the other person would have to be worthy of our forgiveness.

How can I forgive someone who was an asshole to me?
How can I forgive someone who betrayed me?
How can I forgive someone who withheld their love from me?

I felt this way for a long time. If someone "wronged" me, they did not deserve my forgiveness. In fact, the angrier I got, the more I felt I was punishing them.

I quickly realized just how backward this thinking is, however. Getting angry and then angrier was only harming me because it felt like crap. I was the one who continued to hold anger in my body. And I would only get angrier if I felt the person I was angry with didn't "get it" or was not "sorry enough" or sorry at all.

There are a few things I would like to unpack here that I believe will be life changing if you allow yourself to really understand conscious forgiveness.

1. We do not forgive for the other person's benefit. We forgive to liberate ourselves.
2. Having something to forgive means there is something within us that needs healing.
3. Anger means we are judging someone else.

Let me explain.

1. Forgive to liberate yourself

I talk a lot about thinking of our bodies as energy because they *are* energy. Our emotions hold a certain energetic vibration to them. We know this fact because we can feel the difference in our bodies. Having loving thoughts feels different from having angry thoughts. Which one feels better? Let's do a little exercise together.

Close your eyes and think of someone or something you really love right now. Bring that energy into your body. Feel it in your heart center. Breathe that loving energy even deeper into your body. Let it surround you and fill you as you relax into that energy. You might see colors associated with this feeling. Do this for a couple of minutes.

How did that feel?

It probably felt really good. Some of you may have actually felt the vibration of that in your body. It might have felt like goosebumps or electricity or light. Maybe you even smiled. Love feels good because it is a high vibration.

Now let's do the same with anger.

Close your eyes and think of someone you are angry with (either currently or from your past). I want you to really crank up the dial on that anger. Remember what they did to make you feel so angry. Bring that emotion into your body. Take a couple of minutes to really feel it.

How did that feel? What came up for you? What were you thinking?

It probably felt awful. Maybe you literally felt your heart ache or you felt it in the pit of your stomach.

> **RESET: ENERGY CLEANSE**
> 1. Let's reset the body now and do what I call a body sweep.
> 2. Take your hands and, with your intention, sweep from your shoulders down to your fingers, from the top of your legs down to your toes.
>
> Sweep across your heart and neck, then sweep the top of your head, all with the intention of sweeping the anger out of your energy field. You can sweep with crystals or essential oils to help. You can also visualize the color purple, as it is a transmuter color that will help cleanse negative to positive.

When we feel anger and resentment, we literally take our bodies out of alignment. We create disharmony in our energy fields. The longer we hold on to it, the more disharmony we create. The stronger the hate and anger, the stronger the energy that takes us further out of alignment. When we do this long term, it can manifest in our bodies physically.

When we forgive, we let go of these negative toxic energies. We let go because it was ours to let go of in the first place. We are not harming the other person by not forgiving them. In fact, we create great long-lasting damage to ourselves by holding on to toxic energy such as anger, resentment, shame, jealousy, etc.

I know it is easier to say than to do. I have been there, and I still work on it daily, as I realize now that I am worth it. I do not want to feel those negative emotions or bring that energy into my body.

That is not to say we are never going to get mad at someone else or be hurt by their actions, but the question is: How long do you want to linger in that pain?

I believe, as humans, we need to express ourselves and say, "Hey, that hurt my feelings when you did this . . ." or "This made me feel . . ." We express ourselves because we do not want to harbor any feelings, but it is not our job to process or assimilate this information from the other's point of view. That is their job.

We let go of expectations and we say our piece, with love and kindness, and release.

One of the lines I always use to help me shift is: "I get to do me, and they get to do them."

I will tell you how I feel; I need to have a voice, and so do you. But it also means I need to let you be you. If you react badly to what I say or in a way that doesn't satisfy me, then I need to look at what needs to be healed within me. I need to take full accountability.

WTF? Right. How do I take full accountability? Well, that leads to the second part of forgiveness.

2. Forgiveness is a signal for needing healing within

I have worked on conscious forgiveness for a very long time. I know I would not be where I am today or have the relationships I have with my soul family (close ones) if I didn't really work on it. But it still comes up from time to time and means there is some unpacking for me to do, because if I am being triggered by something, then there is something I need to look at.

A couple of months back, I got so hurt by something my husband did. At the time, I thought he was insensitive and a total ass. (I love you, honey!) I was teaching a course to a group of women, and we were unpacking some very delicate issues online via Zoom, which is harder to do and took me some time to build the circle of trust. As a joke, my husband and some of the neighbor kids threw snowballs at my office window, assuming I was done. He didn't think to send a text or consider the fact that I may not be finished. This interruption disturbed my flow, and I felt it was one of my least successful workshops. I felt like he sabotaged my work. My hurt quickly turned to anger when he did not apologize for his actions. Then my anger turned to rage. As the days went on, I kept getting angrier and angrier because I realized I was also mad at myself. I had worked for so many years on how to not hold a grudge, as I did not want that energy in my body, and yet, I was having a hard time letting it go.

The only way I could shift through this situation was to:

1. Express my hurt and vulnerability, and
2. Look at what it was triggering in me. What did I need to learn? What did I need to heal within me?

The truth is, I would not have been so upset if there wasn't some wound I needed to look at. I had a choice that night; I could have brushed it off or made light of the situation. I could have even perceived it as funny and joked about it in my class. But instead, I took it badly and felt like I failed the group. Even though my husband's intentions were not to hurt me, I felt betrayed and overlooked and like my work wasn't important.

After some time and reflection, I realized that what I needed to look at was my drive for perfection; how I beat myself up and shamed myself when and if something didn't go perfectly; how I held myself to such a high standard that was impossible to achieve. I needed to bring some levity and laughter into my business and life.

Wow, this was a lot of unpacking. I understand my drive for perfection was drilled into me as a kid. I am grateful for that as it has made me the ambitious person I am today. The downside (and the part that needed healing) is when we, as ambitious people, beat ourselves up or never feel good enough. My husband's actions had unintentionally triggered my own insecurities of not being good enough. I felt like I hadn't delivered a perfect workshop, which meant my students wouldn't see value in or like me. Moreover, what was I doing to sabotage the workshop myself?

I needed to use this different lens and perspective to assess this event. It was the only way for me to shift from rage to upset to understanding to compassion for myself, and yes, ultimately, to forgive my husband. The true healing journey is in forgiveness but also using the mere fact that you need to forgive as a signal of something needing healing within. To really embrace the truth that everything we witness or are a part of is because it is exactly what we needed; it is always divine intervention and an opportunity for growth.

💡 Write down these three questions:
1. Who do I need to forgive in my life right now? Who am I holding a grudge against?
2. What was it that made me mad? Why was I triggered? Try to get detailed here.
3. What inner reflections can I take from this situation? What blessings did this situation provide for me?

Guaranteed, the first two questions are easier to answer. Simply writing down your answers and getting them out on paper will help with the healing journey. In many instances, we just replay certain experiences, words, thoughts, and interactions over and over in our head, and we turn up the volume on hate each time we do it. When we write things down, it is a cathartic experience because we are releasing it onto paper, something tangible where we can look at it in black and white and start to unpack the lesson.

Question three is harder, but it is where the deeper inner work comes in. This is where we can heal. I promise there is always a blessing in the situation and a learning moment for you, otherwise you would not be angry, and you would not need to forgive. When we are in alignment with who we truly are, we cannot hold on to the energy of anger. It is impossible. Trust this process and do a couple of deep breaths and see what comes to you in answering the third question. The greatest shift can come here and eventually you will get to a place of gratitude because it was exactly what you needed. It is all part of our divine path, even when it hurts.

Mindset shift to help with forgiveness: This is happening for me not to me.

Learning to forgive is actually being able to get to a point when you can view a particular situation or experience as a blessing. The trigger means you are ready to grow; you are ready to transcend, if you choose.

I say again, we are powerful beings who always have choice. The question is, *what* are you choosing?

3. Hating means you are judging

Let's take this one step deeper. This is what I like to call the "inner work" or some of the heavy lifting in personal development.

If I need to forgive you, it means I have judged you. When I hate you and judge you, I hate me and judge me.

This one is harder, but let's unpack it.

When I was angry at my husband, the thoughts going through my head were not very nice:

You idiot, how could you be so stupid and unthoughtful?

Wow, your lack of judgment is something to be admired. (sarcasm)

I don't know you as well as I thought, and you are weak because you couldn't apologize.

JUDGMENT with a capital J. All of it is my judgment of him and his actions. Hmm, if only I could have seen that at the time. Instead, I needed to call a friend and have her sympathize with me so I could feel even more justified in my anger. I needed to punish my husband by not talking to him for a week.

If I had taken a step back instead and looked at his intentions and realized that he had made a mistake, perhaps we wouldn't have had a week-long conflict. But I couldn't because I was so thick in judging his judgment call, or lack thereof, on the situation.

Instead, we need to take the time to step back when we are being triggered and ask ourselves: What needs to be healed within me, and how am I judging this other person and projecting onto them?

Some of the most heartfelt and powerful stories are the ones when we see people forgive what we would think is unforgivable.

I remember going to a powerful talk by a young woman, Amanda Linhoudt, who survived the most tragic kidnapping in

Somalia. You could hear a pin drop in the room as everyone was captivated by her story. She had the most brutal offenses done to her and was tortured in ways that are unimaginable. But the whole message to her story was about forgiveness. She talked about how each morning she makes a conscious choice to point her feet toward the path of forgiveness. Although difficult at times, she said this choice was her path to liberation. She also went on to say that she could not begin to imagine the life her captors lived. They lived in war and poverty from the time they were born. "Who knows how that would affect any of us," she said.

There was not a word from the audience, just tears streaming down most faces as we listened to the captivating message.

There are not many talks that leave that kind of imprint on me and with such a powerful message—a message of forgiveness as a healing power, which we all have and can choose.

Having compassion and understanding to forgive means acknowledging that we all have wounds. We all have a story.

When someone is mad at you or says something mean or does something awful to you, the easiest reaction is to withhold your love, to get angry, and to distance yourself emotionally and physically. And, at times, you need to do it to have space. But for how long? That is when you must work on forgiveness.

What I have also learned is that if I need to heal something as a result of feeling triggered by something or someone, and if someone else in my life is triggered by my actions, the same rules apply to them too.

This has helped me with forgiveness on my own healing journey. Many people were angry with me when I made choices to live in my truth. To leave an unhappy marriage. To marry a man with three kids. Many people in my life at the time were angry that I meditated, did yoga, and was into personal development. I'll never understand why or how someone could be angry about that. I wasn't hurting anyone with my daily practices or my personal life choices. But the truth is if they were so deeply triggered by my simple request to have the freedom to live my life and choose happiness—choose me first—perhaps it is because they hadn't made their happiness a priority. And me living my life shed light on that wound. Chances are me choosing myself reminded them about all the times in their life when they chose to repress their own joy and happiness.

Here's a truth: **We can only be truly happy for others when we have made our own happiness a priority.**

But the problem with this concept is that it is deemed selfish.

Here's another truth: **The real selfish thing is to not have the capacity to be happy for others because you have not had the capacity to choose that for yourself. You become a martyr and**

victim of this life in thinking it is the selfless approach, but really, it does not give you the capacity to embrace others.

We can look at people's reactions at times, and they can seem so outrageous. Like the punishment doesn't fit the crime. The reaction seems so over the top or their anger can seem monstrous. In times like these, I have found it helpful to sit back and take a breath rather than react in the same way. There is one rule in this life that we all have: freedom of choice, freedom of how we react, freedom of how we internalize events and let them either hold us prisoner in our own mind or choose to liberate. Forgiveness is really about liberation and self-love.

We live in a world that is drenched with judgment. We have platforms where people are constantly openly persecuted for their actions or opinions. We have built a society that has become so unforgiving. The reality is that when we judge others, we must judge ourselves first. We see something in the other that we do not like in ourselves. We cannot love with judgment, and we cannot love ourselves when we judge others.

One of my favorite passages and messages from the Bible is the story believed to be about Mary Magdalene (John 8:7): "Let any one of you who is without sin be the first to throw a stone at her."

No one can throw the stone because no one is without sin.

The reality is, we all are figuring out this so-called life that we've been given. We will fuck up from time to time, we will make mistakes, and we will not always get it right. And there will be a time when we will want the grace and forgiveness from someone because of something else we have done.

Forgiveness is one of the hardest things to give at times—it can almost feel painful in our bodies. It is one of the hardest lessons to learn. But I believe that forgiving is really about loving yourself and liberating yourself from the shackles of anger and resentment.

Every time I feel myself judging another, I remind myself of these key points: *Julie, this is not loving yourself if you judge another. Who are you to judge? And what is it that needs to be healed within you?*

And I do know and believe that the more we work on this, the less we have to forgive because we just don't get triggered in the same way. Each time we forgive, we end up healing a part of ourselves that needed healing, closure, understanding, and more. And when we are in love with ourselves—all of who we are—we cannot judge ourselves or others. And when we are free of judgment, we have nothing we need to forgive.

Thank you for the blessing of choosing growth, change, and love.

ME FIRST **means loving yourself so deeply that you can forgive yourself and forgive anyone else in your life who needs it, not for them, but for you—your healing, your inner peace.**

CHAPTER 5

JUDGMENT, WHAT GIVES? SHIFT FROM JUDGMENT TO LOVE

Judgment exists around us and within us—toward everything in our life. Doubtful? Ask yourself if you have been judgmental toward someone today, or even toward yourself?

What can each of us do to be less judgmental and more compassionate? The world needs more love and less hate. Judgment is a form of hate.

The first step is to simply become conscious that you are doing it. Become aware of every time you judge someone else. When you find yourself judging, follow one of the tools in this chapter. The more we practice shifting from judgment to love, the easier it becomes. We create new neural pathways to our brain that are like a reprogramming. But we cannot do that until we become conscious of the fact that we are doing it. If you think you aren't, you are lying to yourself. We all do it.

If you want to change, you can.

> Make a mental note of how many times you judge someone in a day. Big or small, count it out. Each time, ask for forgiveness and send love to that person instead.
>
> Count the next day and the next until you notice the number of times getting fewer and fewer. You will be able to reprogram yourself to judge less often and to be a beacon of love rather than judgment.

The truth is, we all judge. It is inevitable. If you pay attention to your inner dialogue, you will realize that we judge often. Even when we are not conscious of it. Even when we don't want to, we still do. This is a behavioral pattern that has been passed down through the generations, which has become subconsciously imprinted in us as a result. It doesn't help that we witness it in society all the time. We have learned judgment from the time we were young, like a second language. We were taught to judge everything from the clothes people wear, to the different food people eat, to the way people wear their hair, to the actions others take. In fact, we have become an even more judgmental society, as we have different platforms now to express ourselves. We feel called to comment or make an opinion about what people post on social media to how they post it to what they wear and say. However, it has become more hurtful these days because these words now have permanence to them. We can video record or write down our judgments of others, and they are there to stay.

When we were bullied in the school yard growing up, it hurt like hell, but we were able to get over it because once it was done, it was done. People may have laughed and snickered at you, but then they moved on to the next victim until the comments and laughter about you were forgotten. The problem today is that we can revisit a negative remark that someone has posted over and over and over again. This is like a form of torture because every time you read it, you are reprogramming the brain with this energy and reliving the experience time and time again. Your subconscious brain cannot tell the difference between the actual live event and the replay in your mind. So, we are seeing a greater permanent imprint or scarring that happens.

It is okay to have an opinion, but your opinion should be what is right for you. When we superimpose this opinion on others, we are judging them to be less than us or are assuming that our way is better. Better for whom? Them or us? Our way can only be what is right for us. We cannot possibly know what is right for others.

One morning I was out for my morning run, and I was thinking a lot about judgment—about how I could be more mindful and conscious about living with less of it.

Living with the COVID-19 pandemic these past two years has tested this theory of living without judgment, as well as created so many opportunities for growth. For example, over the past two years, I have found myself judging others, especially the government's choices—the level of censorship and the decline of our freedoms and basic rights.

So, there I was, running and thinking about the fact that the best thing for me when I feel the judgment emanating from me is to shift from anger to love. To keep sending love to the government, to keep sending love to the world, as this heals not only myself but also others.

And let me tell you, the universe always helps you when you want to do the deep work. It's almost a *Hey, I saw you thinking about doing deep work; here's an opportunity for you . . . and go!*

So, there I was, running along my usual route, and I passed a lovely lady walking her dog. We waved to each other and said good morning. Moments later, I passed her again on my loop, and I noticed she was holding a cigarette. My first thought: *You are out in nature and getting fresh air with your dog, but you are smoking? I thought you were doing something healthy for your body the first time I saw you, not harmful. Do you realize how bad that is for you?*

And there she is . . . judgment has reared her ugly head.

I laughed to myself as I shook my head. *Well played, Universe, well played.* I was so proud of myself for working on being less judgmental toward anyone and anything, so of course the universe showed me a passerby who I perceived as healthy or someone who makes healthful choices. And how judgmental of me to make that assumption because someone can be 100 percent health conscious AND still be addicted to cigarettes. *Balance. Being human. We all have our vices.*

I laughed to myself, as I got the message loud and clear. We judge each other all the time. It is so easy to judge. Not just others, but ourselves too. And because we judge ourselves constantly, judging others comes to us like second nature.

So, I caught myself at that moment and started to send her love. Love is a great cleaning tool. She was simply mirroring something for me. I used to smoke casually when I was younger.

The thought of doing that now is crazy to me, but there was a point in my life when I did smoke.

TOOLS WE CAN USE TO HELP SHIFT FROM JUDGMENT TO LOVE

💡 **Love Vibes**

I love you, I love you, I love you.
I sent that energy to the woman and myself. *Wow, that feels better.*

💡 **Soap Suds Method**

This method of cleaning is thinking about an image of a really soapy mitt, like the ones you would use while washing your car. Use this visualization to scrub the thought. To clean it. We can do it as soon as the thought arises. Before we even finish the thought, clean it with your soap suds.

Use this technique when you have repeated thoughts around worry or anything you want to change. This doesn't mean we don't feel the emotions that arise with these thoughts, it means we choose to become aware of the thoughts and emotions that surface *and* we choose to honor them and clean them. Eventually, it'll become second nature where you don't think negative, worrisome thoughts.

I think the same method can be effective with judgment.

Use the soap suds method when thinking a judgmental thought, then send love instead. This is a great tool to heal yourself and the world rather than spread more hate.

Forgiveness is powerful. Forgiveness is liberation. Forgiving yourself for judging others and yourself is necessary. Replace judgment with love as often as you can remember. Clean your thoughts as often as you can remember. Begin to develop a different internal program and you will start to see a different experience on the outside.

I'm not sure it is possible to live in a world where you will be completely free of your judgments, but I do know this: You will be provided with many opportunities by the universe to work on it and lead with love instead. Both for yourself and others.

WE ARE THE BIGGEST CRITIC TO OURSELVES

It is important that we pay attention to how often we judge ourselves. We are our toughest critic, and it is this negative self-talk toward ourselves that makes it easier for us to judge others.

Hate attracts hate. And that includes self-hate.

You might be thinking, *But I don't hate myself*, and that may make you feel uncomfortable. But if you are constantly judging yourself, then you are hating yourself rather than loving yourself.

Think about this scenario:

Perhaps you were in a situation where you were either presumptuous, or running late, or couldn't meet the expectations or requirements that were outlined. Chances are your inner dialogue probably sounded like a mix of *How could you be so late?* or *Why can't I ever get this right?* or *Why is it never good enough? Why am I not good enough?*

Your nervous system probably felt alerted in any situation—sweaty palms, racing heartbeat; perhaps you were even trembling slightly. All of this is valid. But it is also a sign that you need to give yourself grace and forgiveness and step out of judgment and into love—toward yourself first.

If you have ever felt judgmental toward yourself or someone else, chances are you also need to judge yourself less, and as always, there is something there within you that needs to be healed. To be seen, heard, felt.

💡 How do you talk to yourself?

Our inner critic can be our worst enemy. The minute you look in the mirror, you criticize all your faults rather than sending love to yourself. Or if you do something wrong, it is so easy to say, "I am such an idiot!" This criticism just becomes so familiar that we do not realize we are feeding ourselves hatred. And the more we do it, the easier it is to engage in negative self-talk, and though it makes us feel like shit, it's like a dopamine hit that our nervous system becomes used to. And when we feel like shit, it is so easy to make choices that are not in our best interest. Like finishing a whole bag of potato chips or a pint of ice cream. Then we feel worse and loathe ourselves even more, thus creating a vicious cycle of perpetual self-hate.

ME FIRST **means looking at** how **you can love yourself more each day.**

Take a step by just telling yourself a few times a day, "I love you" or "I love myself."

You can look in the mirror and say it to your eyes or close your eyes and repeat in your head: "I love myself."

💡 Self-love Mantra

Sit comfortably. Eyes are closed. Shoulders are relaxed. Chest or heart floats.

Repeat:

"I love myself and all my imperfections; I am perfectly imperfect. I love who I am. I have a good heart, and I choose to be happy and wish happiness upon others. Each day I strive to do a little better than the day before. I forgive myself for my mistakes, and I forgive others for theirs. I love me. I love you."

Practice this mantra for one minute a day. Notice how your energy shifts after a week. Notice how you become more conscious of judgments. Notice how judging yourself and others doesn't feel right anymore. Notice how you can change if you choose.

Notice that you always had the power to choose love all along—toward yourself and others.

Promise yourself that from here onward, the negative self-talk will be replaced with loving and kind thoughts, words, and actions.

ME FIRST **means loving yourself and others through the hard moments and choosing forgiveness and kindness—for yourself and others.**

CHAPTER 6

HEALING OUR INNER CRITIC AND LOVING OUR PERFECTLY IMPERFECT SELVES

We cannot talk about self-love, judgment, and loving ourselves without reflecting on how we love our whole selves—every part of who we are. We live in a society that bombards us with ideals about how we should look, eat, sleep, breathe, and move, plus the clothes we should wear and products we should use. You gotta hand it to good marketing—it definitely knows how to make us fall into the comparison trap. And willingly, or subconsciously, we end up falling for it.

Now, not all our negative self-talk toward our bodies stems from the media. As we read in the last chapter, judgment toward others and ourselves comes to us like second nature—and we need to consciously choose to step away from it and move into love.

SELF-LOVE AND OUR BODY

Most women have mastered the art of self-criticism. It has become natural to see faults in ourselves rather than the good. We constantly criticize ourselves, and one of the biggest ways this shows up is in our physical appearance.

Societal pressures to be beautiful according to society's definition of beauty has not helped our inner critic. Social media has us comparing ourselves to so many other people who seem "perfect" with a great life.

Loving our image is not the most important thing in life, but it's an important part of our own healing and self-loving journey. When it becomes easy to criticize our looks, that same critic can easily show up as impostor syndrome when we are attempting to achieve a goal or dream.

So, how do we heal the inner critic that always sees faults in our own appearance? Is the key to care less about it, to accept who we are? Or is it to actually see something different from what we have been masterminding for all these years and convince ourselves of this truth about our flaws?

Aging is an interesting concept. I don't think I thought about my appearance much until I turned forty. Growing up, I didn't really care about my looks, or perhaps I took them for granted. I was more of a tomboy who focused on sports rather than hair dye and nails. Now, to be clear, I don't think there is anything wrong with focusing on your appearance. Whatever it is that makes you feel good, you should do it. But what is sad, and not an act of self-love, is if you only see flaws every time you look in the mirror and you focus your energy on them.

My nose is too big, my nose is too small, these age spots are so ugly, my hair is thinning, my thighs are too big, my body is gross, I am disgusting, I feel like shit, I look like shit.

This criticism has become so easy to do that we don't even realize we are doing it. Every time we hate ourselves, we are creating more unhappiness and dis-ease within ourselves. We are holding that energy in our bodies rather than self-loving energy.

It's time to start reprogramming your inner critic.

The "I Love You" Exercise

1. Make a list of all the things you love about yourself, including your physical attributes.

2. How does it feel—easy or hard? Like anything else, the more you practice this exercise, the easier it becomes. And you start training your mind to compliment yourself rather than criticize.
3. Allow yourself to feel gratitude for all the parts you love and the beauty you see.

If this exercise feels hard, then that is exactly why you need to do it. I want you to get really comfortable with giving yourself compliments. It is typically easier to compliment others than it is to compliment ourselves. And yet the most important message in this book has been about loving ourselves first. So, your inner critic—who has become a master at pointing out your flaws—needs to be healed as well.

Now, every time you look in the mirror, catch yourself. Guaranteed, you will begin to have an internal dialogue about your flaws. Stop and compliment yourself instead. The more you do it, the easier it becomes. The more you train your brain to see your beauty, the less you will see your "flaws." It will take some time, as we have mastered so many years of seeing what is wrong with us rather than what is right.

My family was going out for dinner the other night and my daughter wanted to put on some makeup. As we stood in front of the mirror applying mascara, I looked at her in awe of her beauty. I felt a bit of envy over her body, beautiful hair, and big brown eyes. I wondered if I looked like that at her age and whether she recognized how beautiful she is. Suddenly she began complaining about her eyelashes having a gap. I looked at her as if she were crazy. *What does she see that I do not?* As a teenager, she started to master the inner critic, and how could I blame her when every second Instagram post is on how to have beautiful lashes? It is so deeply ingrained in our society how to perfect our beauty even more. Then, as I looked in the mirror, I saw a million flaws on myself—my skin, my hair, the pimple on my chin. And I realized that I was doing the same thing. Even though I was thinking, *Yah, but my flaws are real and hers are in her head*, I realized that this was such a lie. This was what we keep telling and believing about ourselves.

We have been unconsciously criticizing ourselves from the time we were young. We have been conditioned to care a lot about our bodies and our beauty, and we have become masterful at judging our own flaws. In fact, if we were ever vocal about something we loved about our appearance, we most likely were viewed as a snob or full of ourselves. So, most of us became better at keeping ourselves in check and owning our flaws instead. And, at times, we've even laughed at them because that means we know how to roll with the punches; we've learned to deflect harmful words or thoughts with self-deprecating jokes and comments. Why then give others the satisfaction of judging us or pointing out our flaws when we can simply be our worst critic?

We all have an inner critic to be healed.

One of the things I have become conscious about doing is complimenting people on their beauty. I actually make a point of doing it. I was getting a coffee the other day, for example, and the barista had the most incredible ocean-blue eyes.

I've made a point to really look at people's eyes lately, as most of our faces are covered with a mask, and I believe we need that human connection. I said to her, "Your eyes are the most amazing color; wow are they beautiful!" She blushed and thanked me. I then said, "People must tell you that all the time." She responded, "No, not really."

If we all spent more time vocalizing compliments to people, we would lift their spirits as well as our own. I love telling someone that their outfit looks great or that I like their hairstyle. I think if we could look for opportunities to compliment rather than be critical that we would generally just feel better.

I also look for ways to vocalize appreciation for someone's cooking or their accomplishments at work or the way they dealt with a difficult situation or the way a mom handled a tough problem with her child. But we also shouldn't feel like it is shallow to compliment someone on their beauty. We all have the inner critic about our appearance, so if you can make someone smile by giving them a compliment, why not do it?

HOW LEARNING TO RECEIVE COMPLIMENTS HELPS HEAL THE INNER CRITIC

I have also been really conscious about learning to receive a compliment. About anything. Whenever someone pays you a compliment, do you find yourself shrinking or not wanting to take up space or dismissing it rather than saying thank you? I always did because I didn't want to sound full of myself. The words *Keep yourself humble, Julie* were on repeat in my head.

Learning to receive love is such an important part of the healing journey.

My husband greets me every morning with "Good morning, beautiful." To give you a visual, on most mornings, my hair is standing up on end, my eyes are puffy, and I'm definitely not looking my finest. He has been saying this greeting to me since we have been together, going on twenty years. I realized that most of the time he says it I don't actually hear it. I don't let myself smile.

Instead, my inner voice says, *Yah, right*. But what if I actually let that in? What if I actually leaned into the compliment and allowed it to touch me in a warm way, allowing my beauty to be more than my appearance? What if I allowed myself to heal my inner critic a bit each day with those words?

If we could all point out the good in people and compliment people's beauty as often as possible, I feel we could spread more of that feel-good energy. And if we learn to lean in and say thank you, let the compliment land, and take it in and feel good, we will heal more of our inner critic. Learning to receive love is one of the most important things we can do. Allowing yourself to receive a compliment is allowing yourself to receive that loving energy.

There are always opportunities to compliment someone if you look for them. And every time you do, you will feel better about yourself as well. We can start by looking in the mirror and practicing with ourselves *first*, then look at others and find the beauty that is within us all.

Look at the divine within—you are beautiful. As you are, in your perfect imperfections, because perfect is an illusion. True beauty goes beyond the surface. It means allowing yourself to revel in the beautiful miracle that is your body, your health, your emotions, your abilities, your physical attributes, your creativity, and more! We each have unique traits that make us who we are, yet our humanity is what connects us to each other, so let's celebrate ourselves, let's give and receive love, and let's look for opportunities to always go beyond the surface and love ourselves for *who* we are rather than striving for perfection.

ME FIRST **means learning to receive and give love—to yourself, your body, your soul. It also means celebrating yourself.**

CHAPTER 7

WHO SAYS YOU CAN'T HAVE IT ALL?

It's said that you can't have it all. It's always an either/or. And for a long time in my life, I believed that too. I felt like life was a series of trade-offs and that if you wanted something badly enough, you had to sacrifice something to achieve it. And to an extent, I understand the deeper meaning behind it—there is choice and choosing exactly what to focus on in order to get the results you desire.

However, a large part of our society and the conditioning that runs rampant in it is the belief that you just cannot have it all, all at the same time. Or that "having it all" is for some people—the chosen few, and not you.

I call bullshit on that. I personally believe that we can have it all, but we need to decide what that feels like, what that looks like, then live life in alignment with it. And that often requires us doing this one thing: putting ourselves first.

And no, it isn't selfish to put yourself first. In fact, I'm so glad you're here! It continues to get juicy! Putting yourself first means rewiring your belief system. A great affirmation to start with is:

I AM A PRIORITY

When you repeat this affirmation and then actually begin to believe it, everything will change. You will begin to take what I call inspired action for self-love and care. It will not feel like a chore to love yourself through movement, creativity, connection, food, or whatever other choices feel good, it will just feel natural to you because it becomes an extension of who you are and how you want to feel.

My husband and I were attending a conference with a so-called international guru about how to market your business. The man was hostile and angry. He was angry that more people hadn't shown up to his seminar, and probably for many other reasons.

He was happy, though, to brag about private jets and all the celebrities he had worked with as a coach. I remember sitting in the audience and wondering, *What am I doing here?* I believe time is one of our most precious resources, and over the years, I have become more and more discerning as to whom I spend time with and what I spend time doing. If it doesn't feel right or if it takes me out of my center, I will leave or not commit.

The energy in the room at this conference was heavy; it didn't resonate with me. Before I got up to walk out of the room, the last thing I heard the man say was: "You cannot have it all, so you better pick two things that are important to you. Maybe it is your health and career. Or relationships and money. But you can't have it all, so be willing to choose."

Hearing those words was enough reason for me to walk out. I wanted to grab his mic and tell the audience not to listen to that limiting belief. They shouldn't let this man's wounds impact and influence their beliefs so that they choose their career over the love of their life or compromise their health to succeed.

I know I felt triggered by his words because I used to think like he did. I used to believe it. I used to live that way. Then I realized that this belief system didn't serve me. In fact, it was making me miserable. The only thing that could change was what I perceived to be true. Once I worked on that, things changed for me. I didn't have to compromise my health for my career or loved ones. Remember, a limiting belief is **"I don't have time to do it all."**

We have a picture that we've hung up at our cottage. It has a photo of me and my husband and our blended family of five kids. Below the picture is a quote by Andrea Reiser that says:

"The key to having it all is believing that you do."

I love this quote. Belief has everything to do with it. And "having it all" might mean something different to me than you. But the biggest problem with people not having what they want is caused by the emotional imprints that say you can't have it all, which they have probably heard many times throughout their lives.

So, we approach life from a lack mentality in that we already believe we can't have it all before we even start, which leads us to believe that we have to "sacrifice" to achieve whatever it is we desire. We sacrifice our health or our love for self in order to be a mom or a career woman. We sacrifice our marriages to get ahead. Some of us sacrifice our careers or our dreams to grow our families, have the multiple kids, and the big mansion and two or more cars. We stay in careers that are unfulfilling and drain our energy just so we can have a glimpse of the life we envision. We sacrifice our bodies, our health, and our passions for family or society or even to climb the corporate ladder regardless whether it is our dream to do so. We sacrifice all the time when we make choices. We choose this or that because we believe it is the only way.

And the biggest sacrifice we make is the one to our self. We cannot live our truth or to our full potential if we approach life with limitations and an either/or mindset from the very beginning.

In fact, take a moment to stop and think . . . think about what you truly want.

What is important to you? What do you value? What makes you whole?

Get clear on these answers, as doing so is the most important thing you can do for yourself. Only you get to decide what having it all means to you—other people's judgments can see themselves out the door.

For some people, having it all means having a stable, low-stress job, a consistent paycheck, a decent house to go home to, and a loving partner (and maybe children).

For others, having it all means traveling the world with no commitments to anyone.

For someone else, it might mean being an entrepreneur or

inventor and running a multimillion-dollar company.

And for some, it may be a combination of all of these.

I believe all of it is possible. Where it becomes difficult is when what you believe you want is not actually your belief at all. Meaning, you believe you "should" do it because a) someone told you to, b) you've adopted your family's goals, desires, and values and drowned out your own, or c) you are trying to keep up with the who's who in your community or industry, all of which creates a chase that you become addicted to like an addict who can't ever quite get the ultimate high.

When you are centered and anchored in your truth and believe you already have it all—that is the ultimate high in life.

Not too long ago, I went out for dinner with a really good friend of mine. He is a brilliant man who didn't happen to finish high school. He has created great wealth in his life and also has amazing relationships with the people he loves the most.

At dinner, he turned to me and asked, "Julie, do you really believe it is possible to have it all?"

Now, many people from the outside world might think, *Why does this guy not have it all? He is a billionaire, he shows up to the restaurant in his new Ferrari, and he has a beautiful daughter and wife. What more could you ask for, right?* But I know that none of those things mean that you have it all. That piece of the puzzle must come from within. Nothing in the outside world can give you that. And that is why so many people are always on the chase, the chase to catch something that cannot be caught. To me, peace cannot be caught, it can only be found within.

I thought about his question and said, "Well, I do believe it is possible, but the key to that lies in your own belief system. Why do you keep buying more companies and acquiring more wealth?

What is it that draws you to wanting more?"

He said his wife had asked him the same question. He then answered, "Well I love it and I am good at it."

"Fair answer," I said. "There is no doubt you are working in your zone of genius. You have the remarkable ability to see a company that is failing and to turn it around. You buy companies that are going bankrupt and create success. That is amazing because you make it look so easy, while others look at you and can't understand how you do it. Hence—zone of genius. You found it. Many people search their whole lives in an attempt to figure out what theirs is."

However, that is not the only part of having it all. We have other things that make us whole. And that is why I think my friend asked me the question. Think about it . . .

When we don't have money, we want so badly to make it. We so badly want to have those high-income months . . . or a win at the lottery. We have some type of monetary desire like that.

Yet for many of the people I know who have achieved their monetary goals, once they have the money, they realize it was not a big deal because having money alone cannot make them whole. No matter how much you chase the fast cars, the corner office, the C-Suite jobs, the mansion, and everything else, gaining these things doesn't mean anything if you don't feel whole as you are, anchored into who you are. It all feels meaningless. It feels empty.

So, I went on to tell him to look at the five key areas of life:

Money or Wealth

Career/Purpose

Love/Relationships

Health

Inner Peace or Connection to Source

Because I know him well, I said to him, "You get an A++ on the money part. You get an A on career, but you are still trying to figure out your purpose, so this is not complete yet. You have an A+ in love with others in your life but a C with your relationship with yourself. In health, your score is not great. As for inner peace, you are curious about this one and seeking. But all these things are connected in your life. They are all important. When you put the energy into the other areas that need a boost, you will feel more fulfilled. You will feel whole."

He looked at me and said, "Geez, you are bang on, can we analyze you now?"

We both laughed. And I said, "Trust me, I analyze myself every day on this. Because I believe that is our point: to evolve, to be happy, to be peaceful and fulfilled. Not to be empty or miserable."

What I have realized over the years, and in my own training, is that there are a few key points to having it all:

1. You have to believe you can in order for it to ever be true.
2. You have to be willing to really get to know yourself and decide what YOU value.
3. It is only possible to have it all when you are living from your own center or your own truth.

Take a moment to reflect, assess, and evaluate the five areas of your life. Are they in alignment with who you are, your core values, your desires? Or are you living in alignment with others' choices and expectations of you and for you?

When we begin to put pen to paper about what we value and what we really want, we can begin to consciously attract these aspects in our life.

Write down your top three values and what is important to for each of the following:

Health

Relationships/Love (self-love and love for others)

Money

Purpose/Career

Inner Peace / Connection to Source

Having it all doesn't have to be complicated or a pipe dream. It gets to be yours, in this lifetime, when you feel anchored in your truth, in what makes you come alive, in what fulfills you and brings you joy. When you choose YOU first, living in personal alignment feels effortless. Sure, it may not always please others, but that's the whole point. Living your truth will attract the right people, opportunities, and more into your life . . . you just might have it all within this one lifetime when you live life with the mindset of *me first*.

ME FIRST is your permission slip to only choose what brings you joy and carpe diem the heck out of your life, your way, in alignment with your desires and values.

CHAPTER 8

I HAVE NEVER FELT SAFE TO RELAX

Yikes, that makes you think, doesn't it? When was the last time you felt safe to simply loosen your shoulders and relax? When was the last time you relaxed without having a running to-do list constantly taking up space in your mind? When was the last time you felt safe enough to simply breathe and be who you are?

Recently, I was doing a session exchange with a colleague of mine who is also an emotional freedom technique practitioner. This technique is a powerful way to release the emotional imprints that we have within our bodies. Sometimes these emotional imprints are below the surface of what we think is actually going on. If you struggle with chronic pain or have physical symptoms that manifest "out of nowhere," chances are that while there is a scientific explanation for it, there is also a correlation to the trapped emotions within your body stemming from your past experiences or childhood.

Now, here's the thing: There's not one of us who is spared from having these imprints. We have been influenced in our life and we have made decisions based on these emotional imprints, which then form our belief system. Our belief system governs our life; it is the place from where we perceive our truths about ourselves and the world, and it is the place from where we form action and reaction to events and situations. And beliefs are ultimately what drive our choices each day, which then shape our life experiences.

So, this is key: If you don't like what you are experiencing, then you need to examine your beliefs. Look at what you are believing about something to be true and see if there is a way to come back to center and shift your belief around something or someone. The way to change your experience is to first change your belief, which is where so many of us hold our power yet don't realize it.

The second key is to do a deep dive and assess the experience that you want to change and then to understand the underlying belief and where it comes from.

Is it even your belief? Or is it a belief that you have adopted to be true based on influences or events in your life?

So, for me, one of the biggest aha moments was this realization: "I don't feel safe to relax."

It's nuts, right? But I realized in a session recently that in my whole life, I have never felt safe to relax. Why? Because ultimately, "being busy" was what was modeled for me from my grandmother and my parents, even when I was a young kid. And then there is societal pressure that also dictates this same message: "You need to hustle to get ahead," "Money is not made from nine-to-five," "What are you willing to do or sacrifice in your life to get ahead and succeed?"

No one talks about how to be in flow and live in complete alignment with your desires, something that is the opposite of hustle.

I want to get back to hustle versus flow in a minute, but for now I want to dive deeper into the flawed belief that it is not safe to relax because I feel a lot of people can relate to it.

Does this feeling resonate with you? If you asked me years ago, I'd have said no. But if you look deeper and find you identify with any of these next statements, then chances are you don't feel safe to relax either:

- I feel like I need to multitask.

- I am beholden to time; time dictates a lot of my day.
- I feel guilty relaxing unless I'm on vacation.
- I can't sit still or just "be" without doing something.
- My to-do list is never ending and must get completed before anything else.
- I prioritize other people's needs and wants before my own.
- Even when I am "relaxing," my mind is always thinking about what else I need to do or get done.

Do any of these statements sound familiar? This is the "always on, always on the go" mentality that so many of us are cursed with having, especially if we happen to be ambitious with big lofty goals.

The deeper problem for me with relaxing is that it is directly associated with my false belief about my value and worth. The more I do, the worthier I am. The busier I am, the more value I give. If I truly relax, what am I accomplishing? When I am relaxing, what am I achieving?

So, we hustle, we keep ourselves busy, we constantly feel the need to prove our worth to ourselves and the world. We keep the motor running at full speed and ignore the signs that our body and Universe will always provide us if we would just slow down to listen.

💡 **Let's take a breath break**

Inhale through the nose, fill the belly with air, hold at the top. Exhale through the nose, let the body relax, let the mind relax, and let go.
Inhale: I am worthy to relax.
Exhale: I am at peace.

Let yourself enjoy this feeling for a minute by repeating the breath cycle and really experiencing that peace within the body. Let it fill you completely; use this as a touchstone to know that this peaceful, relaxed place is within you at all moments when you want to choose it.

HOW DO WE CHANGE THE EMOTIONAL IMPRINT SO WE CAN LEARN A NEW UPGRADED BELIEF?
THE BENEFITS OF ENERGY WORK

What I realized in my life was that I was using all my tools to help me overcome my limiting belief of *not feeling safe to relax*. I built self-care habits every day: I meditated, I journaled, I used affirmations, and I worked on reprogramming my brain. All of these helped, and I was very aware of my limiting belief of sacrifice to succeed, that I had to always be busy to get ahead, and that it was hard to not "go, go, go," but I didn't realize that my core belief was that I actually didn't feel safe to relax. *Wow, that is big. Not actually feeling safe. Like if you chill, you get kicked out of this unit that has built itself on hard work and sacrifice.* It was a scary realization because it was like finally putting down your shield that you have used your whole life to protect you. And when you drop the shield (which you might not even realized you were holding), you become vulnerable.

So, I do believe in programming and upgrading our thoughts, but it is hard to do. In fact, our mind can be our biggest enemy. We can tell it not to think something, but it goes ahead and thinks those thoughts more often, creating further stress and bad feelings. We desire to change, but we don't know how, so it feels easier to simply stick with the programming we've grown up with and are accustomed to having.

I'm a firm believer in doing what feels right and good for you and allowing more of that in your life. Make yourself a priority and never feel an ounce of guilt about self-care and self-love. Sometimes you need a bigger boost to shift this feeling in your energy fields or subconscious minds.

When we go back to thinking of our bodies as energy, we can connect the dots that a limiting belief can show up as blocked energy in the body or in our energetic fields, as they hold us back. These energetic imprints can be cleansed out of the body and reprogramed out of our minds.

There are many healing modalities that work with energy and have been very effective and have a common theme: to shift the energy that might be blocked in our mental, emotional, and spiritual bodies and thus also shows up in our physical bodies. When I was in my midtwenties and running my first spa business, I got certified in Reiki—an energy healing modality that many wellness centers use as a therapeutic offering. There are also a lot of tribal rituals such as sweat lodges and Ayahuasca that work on a similar principle. Emotional freedom technique is also very effective in removing energy blocks. The reason I really like EFT is that you can do it on yourself at any time. The principle is to affirm the problem or belief that is causing stress and using the key meridians in the body by using a tapping technique that allows you to shift and remove the blocked energy.

I have used the technique with myself and my clients, and the results are incredible. I have seen huge shifts and awakenings happen in people. For me, my tapping session was powerful because not only did it unlock a belief that I wasn't even aware had dictated so much of my life, but I also could tap on this and move it out of my body and hence, my belief system. (For more information on the tapping technique, please visit the Resources section.)

So that was what I did. I literally tapped on the key points in my body, realizing my fear of relaxing by affirming it.

Tap, tap, tap. "I am afraid to relax."

Tap, tap, tap. "Relaxing feels unsafe to me."

Tap, tap, tap. "If I relax, I won't be productive, and if I am not producing, I am not valued."

Tap, tap, tap. "If I relax, I am not worthy."

Tap, tap, tap. "I am not worthy of relaxing."

Tap, tap, tap. "I do not allow myself to relax because that would mean I am not go, go, go, and go, go, go means I am valued by myself and others."

Tap, tap, tap. "It's not safe for me to relax."

Tap, tap, tap. "If I relax, I will not be appreciated for what I accomplish and what I have done." Tap, tap, tap.

This is years of coding and programming. So, to spend an hour tapping the shit out of this belief that does not serve me is well worth my time because I am ready to live by a different program. And sometimes, you might need more than one session, which is okay. Give yourself that grace.

TO SUMMARIZE: HOW TO REALLY LET THE SHIT GO THAT IS WEIGHING YOU DOWN

1. Affirm what the core issue really is. It may take some digging and uncovering of the layers that you carry emotionally. A good coach can help you. However, in order to shift anything, we need to be aware and conscious of it first.
2. Use energy work such as tapping to help clear this block. You will know it's working because you will feel it in your body; it will feel lighter and easier to do. Reprogramming the subconscious mind will also work. You will need to repeat the unlimited belief instead, over and over, and really work on believing it for that to be true. We will go over that more in Section 2 of this book.
3. Practice it in your life. See how it feels. For me, I had to practice *doing nothing* and feeling in perfect harmony with it. If and when it still feels awkward, then tap, tap, tap, or repeat the opposite of the limiting belief in your mind instead to help shift your energy.

Some things cannot be rationalized or talked away, as sometimes we need a deeper shift. Have you ever noticed that if you keep talking about a problem, it doesn't get better or feel better? In fact, sometimes it feels worse because you keep circling the energy in your mind and body without actually shifting it. Energy is emotion, and emotion is energy in motion. If our words, thoughts, and actions aren't congruent with moving old energy out, we stagnate, our bodies stagnate, and our environment and mindset stagnate. Some people go to therapy for years and talk about the same problems over and over. Now, I am not knocking therapy or therapists, as some people have found it useful and helpful. But for me, I know we have so many layers to unpack in this lifetime that once I become aware of a limitation or belief that does not serve me, I don't want to spend years unpacking it. I personally just want to let it go so I can keep evolving and growing and increasing my threshold on happiness.

Because here is one thing I can promise you: Once we elevate to another level, there will be more limitations that come into our consciousness that we will be ready to look at and release. However, I do believe this is a layered effect. So, if we keep talking about the same problems for years and repeating the same patterns, it is very difficult to ascend to another level of happiness, liberation, and mental freedom, which is everything!

Action keeps you moving. Repeating yourself over and over keeps you stuck. What is meant to help you heal, inadvertently keeps you stuck. Energy needs to move out of your body. Therapy is the gateway that helps you uncover and even get to the root of trauma, yet the way we shift out of this trauma is cultivating safety in our bodies and rewiring our mind and pathways through one small shift at a time, one small action at a time.

What I have learned is that the best thing about taking some time to unpack the layers and identify the core issue is that by dealing with it, it naturally resolves a lot of other problems surrounding that issue. For example, when I dealt with my fear of relaxing, I was able to get into a better flow with my life, my business, and my relationships. I didn't feel like I had to "work so hard" to make it happen. I could actually just be because I was in alignment with my truth, not my limiting beliefs, but my truth. And my truth is that I am worthy of relaxing, I am safe to relax, I don't need to hustle to achieve success, and it doesn't have to be so damn hard. So much of all this was wrapped up in my fear of relaxing.

TRADING THE ILLUSION OF SAFETY FOR HAPPINESS

The other problems that were wrapped up in my fear of relaxing were that I was working hard to nourish and take care of my body with supplements and exercise and meditation but learning to relax was just as important. Sometimes we spend too much time enrolling in all the courses, hiring all the mentors, doing all the right things designed to help us evolve, but we don't actually take the time to be, to breathe, to integrate. In fact, I think not relaxing fully was blocking all the other benefits I was "working so hard" to achieve. There were times I felt drained, and I looked like I was aging so quickly even though I took such good care of myself. I did so much—all tied to the core fundamental problem of it not feeling **safe to relax, which really was not feeling worthy to be able to relax.**

Self-discovery is a powerful process that takes commitment and perseverance. Sometimes I feel like if I lived a more ignorant life, it would be easier because it would not require all this unpacking and self-development. I could just ignore the internal messages. The truth is, I know that it would make me miserable. I knew it at twenty-six years of age when I walked away from my marriage and my previous life with all the safety and comforts built around me. I knew then that if I didn't explore this deep well called self, I would be safe and could stay put. But the feeling of safety was an illusion because I was ignoring myself, I was ignoring my inner voice, I was ignoring my truth. So yes, ignorance might be easier for you; I know it would have been easier for me because there would have been a lot less turmoil with the relationships in my life if I'd stayed put, but I would have also been miserable. So, will you trade the illusion of safety for happiness? I think so many of us don't take risks or leaps in our lives because it feels unsafe, it feels uncomfortable. Stretching out of our comfort zone feels unsafe. Thus, we stay put, we don't grow, we don't listen to the messages that are constantly being sent our way, all for the illusion of safety.

I realized that the trajectory I was on previously was to stay small and stay safe.

On my journey of self-discovery, which is really another word for the choice to love yourself unconditionally, it is your choice to unpack all the things that don't serve you, then look them dead in the eye and say, "No, this belief is holding me back, and it is not even mine. It is a belief that I adopted from someone else who ultimately also adopted the same belief through an experience or event or another person's belief . . . " You then end the cycle that continues to repeat itself.

True freedom occurs when we have the courage to break the cycle, to liberate ourselves, to face our problems, and to get to the root of what is really going on—the core issue—and then look it in the eye and say, "I am ready to release you, I am ready to elevate, I am ready to grow and continue to live an inspired-filled life rather than be miserable and safe."

I had the courage to take this leap, to make the change, but I still carried with me the beliefs from my past of not feeling safe to relax—that I would be judged if I didn't work hard enough, if I didn't sacrifice enough. Over the years, I have been so aware of not wanting to do this, of making huge efforts around my boundaries and my self-care, but the belief was still in my energy field. Awareness is key, but so is integration, which is why I do believe energy work is an amazing healing tool to help us release, let go, and liberate ourselves.

Start choosing yourself first. Choose to break the cycle. Choose to cultivate safety within your body by breaking free of the societal pressures and norms that don't serve you or elevate your life. Growth and change feel uncomfortable, but so does staying in the same place or circumstance year after year. Much of that can shift with a small shift in your beliefs, how you love yourself, and what you choose to be, do, think, and act upon every day.

ME FIRST **means feeling safe enough to be who you are.**

CHAPTER 9

WORKING FROM A PLACE OF INSPIRATION VERSUS HUSTLE

Work hard and you will get ahead.
Money isn't made nine-to-five.
You have to sacrifice to make it in life.
Nothing comes easy.
You need to be prepared to do what others aren't willing to do.

I lived by these beliefs for most of my life.

Growing up, I did not know what a Saturday night dinner at

home felt like with the family. I have absolutely no memory of one because it did not exist. In fact, the only night we had dinner together as a family was Monday.

I cherished Monday nights growing up because both my parents were home and the whole family was able to enjoy a meal together.

I may sound biased, but I have to say that I think my dad is one of the greatest cooks in the world. However, as a young kid, I didn't necessarily appreciate it because I just thought it was normal to eat like we did. It wasn't until my friends came over for dinner and piled their plates with food and went on and on about how good everything tasted that I thought, *Well, doesn't everyone eat like this?*

Then, when I went off to university, I lost fifteen pounds because I thought the food was inedible. Instead of gaining the "freshman fifteen," I was the skinniest I had ever been.

It made me realize I was privileged to have so many things in life and that I was grateful for all of them: amazing food, private school education, opportunities and connections, working from a young age and always having a job (this was a blessing and a curse).

But the one thing I was not privileged to have was time: time for the simple pleasures in life. Time with my parents, time to sit together as a family and watch movies or play card games, time to go for evening strolls or to watch a sporting event together, time to see my parents cheering at the sidelines while watching my basketball games. Time was the limited resource in our family, and I realize that this fact is what has contributed to so many of my limiting beliefs around time.

My parents, like many, immigrated to Canada when they were young. They came from poverty and worked hard to support their families. My mom, at a young age, had to fight to stay in school because my grandmother wanted her to work to help pay the bills.

In reflection, we are influenced so greatly by our upbringing, which shapes our belief systems. When you can look at the circumstances that shaped an individual and what contributes to their core values, you can understand them on a deeper level. I know that for me, this perspective has helped me so much on my healing journey.

For my parents, their driving force was providing for their kids and creating a "better life." They would do it at all costs because they wanted to break free from the cycle of poverty in their lives. Thus, my mom valued education because she had to fight for it herself. And both my parents valued hard work because that was how they proved to get ahead in life and provide for us.

So, my parents are the perfect contributors (and for good reason) to the term "hustle."

In fact, I feel like they perfected the work and hustled in a way that I didn't think was humanly possible. They worked, on average, seventeen-hour days, almost six or seven days a week. Growing up, this schedule was the norm. This is what it took to "get ahead."

We were in the hospitality industry, an industry that has demanding and unsocial hours. When everyone else seemed to be enjoying life, we were the busiest. Weekend days were the longest days of the week.

I remember being about ten years old when I first started working in the kitchen beside my dad at our banquet hall, peeling carrots, chopping onions, and wiping out ashtrays (yuck). As I grew older, especially around fourteen, I was so jealous of my friends, as they were able to go to the movies on the weekends or up to cottages, while I had to work. I remember feeling it in the pit of my stomach when I felt left out. I remember thinking, *Why do we have to work so hard and others don't?* Yup, we learn how to compare and despair at a young age.

Whenever I tried to talk to my parents about my schedule, I was quickly shut down. My siblings and I were told to never complain and to instead be grateful that we had a business that provided the lifestyle we enjoyed. But even at that young age, as it was normalized for me to hustle and work way more than play, I remember thinking, *But what lifestyle is this providing when we don't have time to even go for a walk together or play a game of catch?*

We did have the privilege of taking a family trip together over spring break on most years. And yes, there was a lot of gratitude for these trips, and it was ingrained in us that these were rewards from working so hard. So, the work/reward ratio was indoctrinated in me at a young age, and it was normalized that you worked many hours to be rewarded for very few hours of leisure or travel.

In my first job out of university, I was determined to break free from having to work every weekend of my life. So, I took a stab at the corporate world. I got my first job as a business manager at a bank, lending to the small- and medium-sized business sector. I thought, *This is my ticket to happiness. I get my weekends off for the first time in my life. I have a great job with decent pay, and I can have a comfortable life.* A life, to me, meant having my weekends off. I could finally enjoy the lifestyle that all my friends had growing up and that I envied. I was newly married, we had bought our first home, and we lived in the city in a very hip area that was walking distance to great shops and restaurants. Life was amazing, or so I thought.

It wasn't until very shortly into my job that I realized I hated it. I hadn't even finished my training. The people I worked with were amazing, but I hated the whole bureaucratic environment. I felt like a trapped animal, like I had to just follow rules and regulations and had absolutely no room for creativity. I looked at the "lifers," those who had spent their whole careers there and had climbed the corporate ladder, and I thought to myself, *I have no aspiration to be you.* And as an ambitious person, I also remember thinking, *What is wrong with me? Why do I not aspire to be them?*

My job was to assess small- to medium-sized businesses that were looking for finances to either expand or start new businesses. As I met my clients and assessed their businesses, I remember looking at them across the desk and wishing I could trade places. I realized really quickly that I was not a banker; in fact, I realized that I was not cut out for the corporate world—I'm an entrepreneur.

Despite the modeling for me that being an entrepreneur meant you had to work like a dog, anything was better than the rigid corporate world. I was not able to be in my own flow or tap into my own creativity. Rather, I had to wait to get deals approved based on risk-management timelines. I had to follow form and had no free flow in my job at all. I hated it, but I was not a quitter.

So, I stuck it out for a year. In that year, my body screamed at me in every way to wake up and listen. I started having panic attacks. I had never had a panic attack in my life, and it felt like I was having a heart attack. I got hooked up to every machine possible to monitor my heart, and everything came back clean. I remember saying to my doctor, "But you don't understand. I think there is something seriously wrong with me." I worked out, I ate healthful foods, and I was young. WTF?

The doctor told me that stress can show up in many ways in our body, and that panic attacks are common for people who are under a lot of stress. But at that time, the only thing I felt stressed about was my job. And not the job itself, but the fact that I didn't like it. In fact, I prayed that I would get a really bad cold so I could call in sick. I only did that once and felt guilty as heck because there was no such thing as "calling in sick" while I was growing up. You took your vitamins and got your ass to work. But it made me realize how powerful the mind-body connection really is. My body was literally revolting over my life until I was willing to have the courage to look at it.

So, I stuck it out for a year and then gave my notice.

I didn't have a panic attack again. I chose to make the changes in my environment and listen to my body.

So now what? I finally had my weekends off, I was working decent hours, then my body revolts and has panic attacks. What did this mean? I was working less and suffering more. I was so confused.

What I did next was take the word "hustle" to a whole new level. I realize now that doing that was what was familiar to me—that was what felt safest.

At twenty-three years old, I went from the corporate world to the wellness world. At the time, my family was talking about adding a spa to our resort business. We had skiing, golfing, weddings, and corporate events, and we felt a spa would be the right complement to the business.

My mom, who was running the family resort business, approached a spa consultant to help her. She was a leader at the time because spas were still a new thing in Ontario resorts. For most, they were an afterthought that was then put in the basement. My mom quickly realized that to do it right, it would take millions of dollars in expansion, but she began the process. There were not many people with experience, however, so the consultant asked if anyone in the family would be interested in being trained. My mom approached me, and I thought it sounded interesting. I have always been passionate about wellness, so I took the leap.

I hustled my ass off, but the difference was that I loved the work, and I felt a passion that I never felt while in the corporate world. I was learning about drawings and construction and spa equipment orders, by day and by night, and I was in school earning my esthetics diploma. I was putting in seventeen-hour days and working seven days a week. This was normal; this was what I was familiar with—this was my upbringing; this I could thrive in.

I was back on the grind but felt a weird sense of relief because it was familiar, and I loved it. It felt safe and exhilarating at the same time. I was working seven days a week to turn this dream into a reality and make my hardworking parents proud. I thought the only way to do it was to work harder than they did, something that was not easy to do, but I did it. I put my head down and learned everything there was to learn about the spa world. I conducted my first interviews and hired and managed a team of fifty employees. I was initiated by fire. "No" was never an answer, I just had to figure it out and make it happen because as an entrepreneur, that is what you do.

Hustle, hustle, hustle, and if you don't know the answer, you figure it out.

After a year of the hustle, we had record numbers, I cracked seven figures in revenue in a year, and we had five-star customer reviews. I was kicking ass and my belief system of "you have to sacrifice to get ahead" was drilled even deeper in my head. So, I missed friends' birthdays, holidays, walks in the evenings, spending time with my husband, going out for dinner, etc. *So, I missed all of this, right? But I was kicking ass in business, so it was worth it, or what I was supposed to do. So I thought....*

But then a restless stirring began. Again. It was as if the pendulum had swung in the opposite direction, but I was still so out of balance. I liked my work, but I knew my schedule wasn't sustainable. And things started to come out sideways because I lost perspective on life. I was so caught up in my own little world that nothing else seemed to matter.

I believe life will kick you in the ass until you get back to your center. The way I was living was not sustainable. The level of hustle was insane, even for a New York stockbroker.

I remember driving to work on Saturday morning with my cousin, a teenager at the time, who worked at the spa for her summer job. She could sense that I was off and asked me what was wrong. I told her about an aesthetician who quit and how I was so upset about it.

She turned to me and said, "Well, maybe things feel like a bigger deal to you than they actually are because all you know is this spa. All you do is work; this has become your life, so when something goes wrong, it feels like such a big deal because you have no balance in your life."

A lightbulb moment.

I looked over at her and wasn't sure if I should feel annoyed because she triggered a truth button for me or be impressed with her wisdom and perspective at fifteen years old.

She was right. I had no perspective, and this was no way to live life. The turning in my belly began. I knew my lifestyle wasn't right for me, and I knew it could not be how the rest of my life played out because truthfully, I wasn't happy. I was only fulfilling one piece of me, and it was way out of whack.

And so it all came crashing down, because it had to. It blew up like a volcano, because it had to.

I was not living my truth; how could I even know what that was? And I surely wasn't living from inspiration but from my memory of "work your ass off."

How does one break free from this cycle of hustle? I actually hate the word hustle. I know it is commonly used in the entrepreneurial world, but I honestly hate the energy around the word and what it represents.

What if we could go from hustle to inspiration? Hmm, is that even possible?

Today, years later, after much work on my own limiting beliefs and helping others with theirs, I realize some key things about success.

> *You have nothing to prove in this life to anyone but to live your life.*
> –Don Miguel Ruiz, *The Four Agreements*

When we work from inspiration, we notice some key things:
- It flows.
- It feels easy.
- It doesn't feel like work.
- You can be really efficient at it (it doesn't have to take all your time).
- It fills your heart.
- You feel whole.
- You succeed without sacrificing yourself.
- You get ideas that you couldn't possibly think were possible.
- You nourish all the parts of your life because you realize it is all connected.

When we work from hustle mentality or the limiting belief of sacrifice to succeed:
- It feels hard.
- It is always out of balance.
- You work from a place of "I need to, I should do. I don't have time for this or that. . . ."
- Other key areas of your life inevitably suffer: your love, relationships, health, etc.
- Life passes you by.

Today, when I work with my clients, the first place we start from is the place of desire. Think about the following question:

💡 What do you want in your life?

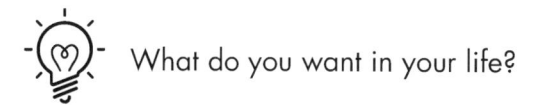

This is the hardest question for people to answer.

But when you can marry up desire and passion with purpose and career, it is magic. It is what we all deserve—to really be courageous enough to do what we were meant to do, whatever that is, and not what we were told to do.

The doing is important. But the doing, when it comes from inspiration, feels fantastic. You feel inspired to do it rather than dragging your feet or trying to convince yourself that this is what you need to do so suck it up and get it done.

I believe that everyone can work from a place of inspiration in their life. You can work from a place of flow. But first you have to get to know yourself intimately; you need to uncover your desires like opening a special gift that you have been waiting for. You need to set free and be comfortable with being who you really are and who you are meant to be, not who you are told to be. For so many, we stop at that point because it either feels scary or we have too many messages that have created weeds in our gardens that then choke out our bright flowers, not allowing them to bloom.

The saying that life is a journey is so true. Every day is part of this beautiful journey, and each one can feel like heaven, or perhaps hell. It truly is what we make of it. The road on our journey takes turns and bends, it has bumpy and smooth paths. This journey will give us all the experiences that we need in order for us to grow into who we really are.

The journey of life can be the journey to our authentic selves. Many may never actually uncover their truth or have the courage to live it. For others, they need numerous twists and turns on the road before getting there. And others understand and get it from a young age and have such a strong sense of self that nothing will sway them.

> Where are you on your own journey? Are you at a bend? Is there a clear vision ahead or does it look cloudy?

I believe that the inner work of discovering your truth is the most important work you can do. For some of us, this requires deeper work or more peeling back of the layers than for others.

You are worth it!

Because this is your destiny; this is your path to freedom and liberation; this is how we achieve heaven on earth.

The first step to getting to a place of inspiration is finding your truth.

ME FIRST **means having the courage to uncover your truth and to live it wholeheartedly. Living your truth will set you free.**

CHAPTER 10

WHO AM I TO DO THIS, DESIRE THIS, BE THIS?

Beware of the impostor syndrome; at some point, it hits us all.

I remember a time when it was cloudy outside, and the air was thick with humidity. Everything just felt heavy. That must be why I felt so emotionally drained. I felt stuck; I had a hard time grounding my energy. In fact, I felt insecure. *Who am I kidding? It has nothing to do with the thick air outside.*

But I find it easier to blame something or to come up with a reason as to why some moments or days just feel harder. When we look to the outside world for our answers about why we might be feeling inadequate or frustrated, it is much easier because it helps us avoid looking at the inner truth, which then creates vulnerability.

Heavy messages include: *Who am I to want more in my life? Who am I to think I have anything to offer others? I am not worthy of (fill in the blank).*

IMPOSTOR SYNDROME

Impostor syndrome is something often heard of within the entrepreneurial and professional world—I think we all have it in moments, but we keep it hidden, we keep it quiet, or we try to bury it. When we try to bury our emotions or are not honest with our feelings or avoid leaning into the emotion to discover what is beneath it, we can never truly heal. It is impossible to feel carefree. Burying or ignoring it makes us feel heavy and dense. And as we bury it over and over again, we will accumulate more heaviness, more denseness, and more thickness in the layers of the onion. The golden nugget of truth gets harder to find. But it is always there, and if we are brave, we can unpack what we need to and look it straight in the eye to confront the limitation to heal it. Declare it to move it.

I had a powerful session with a client dealing with her impostor syndrome of not being enough. For many of us, this shows up in how we shy away from asking for a well-deserved raise, not charging enough for our services, giving too much of ourselves and then feeling depleted, or not feeling like we have a voice or can speak our truth. All these things are complex yet simple messages that we have had on repeat in our heads. But even if we want to change it, it can be super frustrating because as much as we may want to let it go, it keeps rearing its ugly head. It holds us back and shapes our lives in more ways than we realize.

The feeling is so real that it can feel suffocating or intolerable but normal—"normal" because it is so familiar. For many of us, like my client, we can realize this stems from a long time ago when we inherited a belief about the world or others that impacted our beliefs about ourselves.

So, how do we deal and how do we heal? Are we doomed forever?

When we are ready to face the core issue of what lies beneath the surface of our impostor syndrome, we can move this blocked energy, imprint, or belief from our body.

My client was having a difficult time asking for a raise. She knew she was being paid less than her colleagues, and yet she was managing a bigger portfolio. Impostor syndrome held her in place by saying, "Yah, but look at what you are making, and you don't even have a degree. You are lucky to have this job, so don't fuck it up by asking for more. Stay in your lane."

And on and on, these are the stories we tell ourselves even though we know it doesn't feel good. They weigh us down and are so familiar. In many ways, these messages keep us safe because they keep us small. They allow us to be okay with where we are and not ask for more because the fear of rejection is so big. If I stay quiet, I don't get a no; therefore, I keep the peace.

LOOK your shit right in the face to shift:

There is always something below the surface. It is not about asking for a raise or even about money but rather the time in your life when you decided that you weren't worth it.

Uncovering the core issue:

Question: "When was the first time you can remember feeling this way?"

Client: "As a kid, sitting at the dinner table, I never felt like I could have a voice. Everyone else was loud and took up space. I decided it was easier to be quiet."

Response: "So, at the time as a kid, you imprinted the belief that your voice doesn't count, does not carry weight. And you made decisions about this in your life based on this truth you decided."

The key to note here is that you are making this contract with yourself; the people around you who are participating in making you feel this way are not part of your deal. You may want to say it is their fault, but I guarantee you, they had no clue you were making this deal with yourself.

So, now your future self can look at that truth nugget and tap into forgiveness, not only for the people in your life but also for your younger self who believed it to be true all these years and held you back because of it.

Then we flex the muscle that we have kept dormant. We show up consistently, and we take action toward what we want and deserve. One small step at a time.

We exercise this muscle we have kept hidden and quiet for years—the muscle to ask for what we want and deserve. It is never about money itself, it is always about the perception of money and our worth that we connect ourselves to in relation to money. When we see this truth about what it is, we can begin to move it through our body.

Every single one of us experiences impostor syndrome and feelings of not being enough. However, when we anchor into our desires and start peeling away the layers, much like an onion, we can get to the root of why we feel a certain way, why the fear exists within us. And once we uncover that root, we have a choice: to stay the same or to shift and expand into greater consciousness by taking aligned action.

Living in alignment does not mean that it won't be scary or that there won't be challenges. It means that when you are in alignment, you will find a way to keep showing up, keep going, keep asking for what you desire. And as you continue to flex these muscles, living in alignment becomes easier and feeling like an impostor starts to become a shadow you once knew.

It is very common for people to have impostor syndrome around thoughts about money. But as I said, it rarely has to do with money itself but rather our relationship to money and our sense of self-worth. We can heal this imprint and build a new relationship with money and our feelings of worthiness for abundance. This inner work is time well spent because it can take us out of a repeated pattern that doesn't feel good, as well as shift us from a mentality of lack to one of prosperity. When it comes to money specifically, I have found it helpful for my clients (and me!) to understand that money is energy, just like anything else. It is a form of exchange in our world. When we work on our worthiness to receive, it becomes easier to receive more money. It becomes easier to charge our clients what our services are worth. It becomes easier to ask for the well-deserved raise. So, raising your vibration to feel worthy to receive will help you attract more abundance in your life.

TRY SOME OF THE FOLLOWING AFFIRMATIONS TO HELP WITH MONEY BLOCKS:

"I am worthy to receive."

"I give great service and I receive great pay."

"I love money."

"I am prosperous and abundant."

"Opportunities come to me; I am open to receive."

ME FIRST means showing up for yourself no matter what and trusting that who you are is enough. It means that your desires want you just as much as you want them, and it means living in alignment with that. You are worthy of your heartfelt desires.

CHAPTER 11

OUR DIFFERENCES ARE WHAT MAKE US HUMAN

I wanted to scream from the rooftops, "Don't do it!" My stomach ached, and I felt heartache and sorrow as I witnessed so many people I love make decisions I "judged" to be not in their highest and best interest.

I am out of alignment. I am out of my truth because I am in a place of judgment. I own it.

So now what? So much of my purpose is about empowerment. My whole company is built on the principle of teaching people to become the most authentic and empowered version of themselves possible.

I am a hypocrite if I judge others' decisions. They are individuals and have a right to make their choices. This is free will. The minute we take free will off the table, we have lost our fundamental human rights.

I take a deep breath, and I have a good cry. This past year, we have created so much fear and separation within families and communities, local and overseas. I grieve some more over this reality, and I pray. I work on healing the part of me that is in judgment of others; even if it comes from a place of love, I still recognize it as judgment.

So, I continue to heal myself, to clean my energy field that holds these judgments, and I remember a time in my life when I felt ostracized for the decisions I made to follow my truth. It was not deemed as appropriate. I remember how sad this made me feel and unsafe to follow my truth. So, who am I to judge now after I've been there, after I have been judged and ostracized for my choices? We can all justify judgment. We can all say, "Yeah, but . . ." or "This is different . . ." or "This is crazy! How can't you see you are making the biggest mistake of your life?"

Have you ever said something like that to your kid? I bet that it didn't feel good. So why do we say it to ourselves and others? Why can't we embrace our differences and our personal choices and empower each other to live our best lives?

THE PATH TO PEACE

There are two key concepts that help me with my path to peace:
1. We are all on a journey and are here to figure things out. Everything we are faced with is to help us on our journey to grow and to learn and to evolve.
2. We all have the freedom of *choice*. We are free to make our own choices.

So, why do we need to have everyone agree? When we have agreement, we feel more secure about ourselves. It reaffirms that we made the right decision for ourselves, even when a part of us might be hesitant or second-guess our decisions.

Now, what if you could just be at inner peace with yourself? Could you love yourself unconditionally so that you don't need someone else to agree with you and make the same choices as you have to feel whole? What if you just stood strong in your place of knowing yourself so that nothing and no one could sway you from your truth? So that other people's decisions didn't create anger or an illusion of separation within you? So that they are here to be themselves, and you are free to be yourself? How would that feel? To me, even as I write these words and feel them in my body, it feels freeing, expansive, loving, and kind.

I realize that this is the way I want to live and be in this world. I also realize that I have work to do, as the past year we have witnessed an unearthing of issues that need light. We have witnessed mass instances of censorship that have always been there but are now more prevalent and are being brought to light. We have witnessed some of our medical freedom being taken away from us. We have witnessed social shaming due to our medical choices. Yikes. That stings. It really does. And we can still interact with each other with love and kindness at the forefront of each interaction and conversation. Yes, even when it is hard to do that. This is where growth comes in, where awake and aware consciousness comes in, where leading with love and kindness will always win, even when others around you don't understand.

Growth, growth, growth. With every controlling tactic or government policy that came out this past year, I continue to tell myself to breathe, pray, and heal, and that this is an opportunity to lean into trust and stand in my truth.

In the Bible, Genesis 3:19 reads, ". . . for dust you are and to dust you will return." We come from the same place, and we are going to the same place. In my opinion, the Bible is filled with nuggets of wisdom, and we all have a choice about how we interpret it. Therefore, according to this verse, there is no separation between you and me. At the end of the day, we are all human. We are connected through our shared experiences, our humanity—not color, gender, socioeconomic status, political view, education, you name it. Whatever creates an illusion of separation here is not taken with us to the other side when we pass away. To me, this is a profound concept, because when I feel judgment or separation based on belief or opinion, I recall this verse.

So, I breathe into this awareness and a sense of calm is restored, and I can get back to my center. You don't have to agree with me, as this is just my personal interpretation. We are on a path, a journey. We can share opinions and experiences out of love, not judgment. And that is a very different energy and tone.

My husband and I were driving up north one day so I could carve out some time to write this book. I find being in nature helps with my inspiration because it feels closer to the divine to me. I am intentional with this book. I want to write from a place of inspiration rather than forcing it out or trying to hit a deadline.

Then my stepson called, my husband's eldest child. Gosh, I love this kid. We got into a light debate on the phone over a difference of opinion. I am really conscious about leading from a place of love, but I could feel myself getting charged because I care and hope he is making fully informed decisions about his life. Again, I'm balancing the thought of *Who am I to say this?* with my concern out of love and no judgment. I say to him, "I see through things, and it worries me."

After we hung up, my husband said, "Julie, that might have sounded different if you said, 'Well, my opinion is that I feel . . . because ultimately it is my opinion. That doesn't mean it is right or wrong, and it doesn't matter; it is my opinion based on my lens of where I am standing today.'"

Sigh. It sometimes feels exhausting to do the inner work and constantly look at our feelings and learn from these moments. But the fact is that it is my opinion. And I love you—yes, you, the one reading this book—no matter what you do or how you think, which always goes back to intention. If a person's intention behind making a choice—no matter what that choice may be in life, business, health, wellness, love—is from a place of love and wanting to do the right thing, then who the hell am I to judge? Who the hell are any of us to judge?

If we make choices with the intention of harming others, that is another story.

"Thou shalt do no harm."

An intelligent and divinely inspired principle of the Hippocratic oath that feels in alignment with me. Our basic human currency is love.

Do I think there are lost souls? Absolutely. We see that with everyday crimes—troubled souls who have not found the healing they need, which then results in them causing harm to someone else. These actions can only come from a place of feeling harmed or wounded within oneself.

And hence, I refer back to the premise of this book. The most important thing you are in control of, your job or soul purpose, is to heal and love yourself more and more every day. The more we heal, the less harm we inevitably do to others.

When something triggers you or gets you fired up, look at the opportunity it is presenting for you to look within yourself rather than go into blame or shame. Blaming or shaming another creates more separation. We are all human, we are all connected, we are all one. I judge you, I judge me. I shame you, I shame me. I blame you, I blame me.

I love me. I love you.

What matters most is not what happens when we are done living our life here on Earth but what happens in each moment and who we are becoming in each moment while we are still alive and have the privilege of living the life we live.

It is easier to love one another and be compassionate when we shift from judgment to curiosity.

If I change my lens from judgment or separation and see you for what you really are, then I will see a divine being. Your actions and behaviors do not make you more or less worthy of anything. You are already worthy. The key is to just know this fact. I can love you and forgive you when I see your true self.

You are on this path trying to figure it out, just like I am. You are here to remember that you are divine. Choose different experiences that will either get you closer or further from this truth—whatever that feels like for you.

We all want three basic things as humans:

1. Love
2. Safety
3. Belonging

Our actions, however, may be in contrast because we can be on different parts of the journey. But we are still one. We are still connected. We all want the same thing.

LOVE

When we love, we realize that it is our innate human currency. This vibration heals all things. How do we know? Because we can feel the difference of love in our bodies.

When you have hateful thoughts toward someone else, you feel that energy in your body. You are the one who suffers. Think of the last time you were really angry at someone. You might have even wished them harm, and even though you knew it was wrong, you still felt it.

How did that make you feel?

I guarantee you felt like shit because it is impossible to feel good, to feel whole, to feel peace when we hate someone else. No matter what they have done, we feel like shit when we hate.

We are all connected. Love is the only way.

SAFETY

We want safety. We are hardwired for safety. We want to feel whole and safe to be who we really are. To express our unique self. Yes, you are uniquely you, and you and I are different, but we are still connected.

In our society, when we feel threatened about not having freedom of expression or opinion, we do not feel safe. When our basic human liberties are taken away from us, we do not feel safe. How can we live in a universe where we are allowed to have differing views, where we are allowed to express ourselves, and not threaten someone else? The key to this is "to know thyself."

When you are in touch with your own sense of self, your sovereignty, you cannot possibly be threatened by someone who has an opposing opinion. You can get curious about it and ask questions, but the minute you feel yourself judging them, it's time to look within because there is more inner healing work to do within you.

I have learned that when I feel safe to express and be who I truly am, I can remove my judgment of you. So again, it comes back to taking full responsibility for who you are, to be comfortable in your own skin so you can let others be comfortable in theirs, to understand that perfection and right and wrong are an illusion. Instead, it is what is right for YOU. And that same governing rule holds true for others. It is what is right for them. Nobody else gets to make that decision for you. Acting out of our human currency of love leads to the feeling of safety.

BELONGING

Belonging goes back to the tribal days. Having your tribe was sacred. It made you feel part of a bigger picture, part of the community. The true empowerment here is when you realize that you belong no matter what. You belong because we are all connected. We are all divine. But some of us change who we truly are in order to belong. We dampen our inner voice and squash our true essence to fit in.

As a kid, I remember being comfortable speaking in a crowd, dancing without a care, singing loudly, and putting on a show, even if I was tone deaf or bossed around those who I felt needed it. I was confident and unafraid to stand out. But what I realized over the years is that I did this within the boundaries of what I knew I could stretch and with what was comfortable for me. I might rock the boat a bit, but when the water became choppy, I would hide a part of me or shrink myself a little to belong. I think many of us do this for fear of not fitting in and ultimately being outcasted. When we do this little by little over the years, we don't even realize we are doing it. In fact, I believe for most, we lose our sense of self to belong.

What if you could belong and be different? You could be wholly you and be part of your community. Belonging should never mean conforming. But as a society, we have made it that way in order to be accepted. Anyone who stands out is considered "the rebel" or "the black sheep of the family."

Why? Why can't they just be themselves and be embraced for who they are? I think this is the biggest work we need to do, and it starts within. We may have all felt we had to conform, and we may want to blame others for it. That would be easy.

But when we can take full responsibility for our actions and see how and when we dimmed our own light to belong, then we can realize we are the only ones who have the power to change it, to turn our lights back on.

I believe you can belong in your world AND be different. Sometimes it might take time, patience, and a lot of healing to feel it, but love always wins in the end. Unity always wins in the end. Because that is our human design, but no one else is in control of it but you. Working on your own sense of sovereignty is the most important piece in this puzzle. Let this help you know the same is true for you when others make you feel like you don't belong. It is an illusion because we all belong, always. We are all divine beings, and to know thyself means you can never not belong!

ME FIRST **means the more comfortable I am in my own skin, the more accepting I am of you.**

CHAPTER 12

CURIOSITY ALLOWS EXPANSION

Curiosity is something we're born having. Kids are curious with their imagination, and they explore it daily through creative play. They may talk to their imaginary friends or imagine that they are in a fairy land with rainbows and unicorns. They see the world with vibrant colors and a sense of wonder, awe, and magic.

Why do we lose this imagination or curiosity when we get older?

Curiosity is such an important part of being a human being. People tend to get fixated on their beliefs, however, thinking there's no other alternative to what they believe in. And beliefs are a big part of what dictate our lives. Our beliefs govern our choices and decisions, which then dictate our experiences in this life.

Our belief system is the most powerful thing we have, whether that belief system serves us or not. It still dictates how we live. I have witnessed over the years, even with myself, how a belief system can lead someone to misery and unhappiness, yet we cling on to these beliefs because it is what we have been told to do; it is what has been indoctrinated into us.

No wonder it can be so tiring and confusing to be human. Where does freedom come in? How do we find the strength and courage to siphon all the messages we have been told and then find our truth? Find our beliefs that are truly ours, not those of other people? It is especially difficult when some of the messages that are indoctrinated in us come with a dose of fear, guilt, and shame.

We have witnessed time in history when humans have been told what they should and should not do with force and coercion. Fear has been one of the popular guiding forces around messaging throughout history. We have seen belief systems that have caused divides in countries, communities, and families. Even when an inside voice might question some of the narrative, for most people, their fear was way too strong and overruled rational thought process.

So, what does this mean? In a time of world crisis, do we succumb to having a divide in humanity? Do we lose our sense of self even more? Do we lose our individual freedoms that our ancestors worked so hard to gain for us? Do we lose our sense of individuality because we fear being ousted or not belonging with the narrative? Do we lose our curiosity?

Maybe we do. Or maybe we take a path less traveled and listen to our inner divinely guided voice.

However, many people are willing to adopt a belief system if that is what the "higher" powers tell them to do, higher powers being family, peers, colleagues, bosses, the powers that be—in your life, business, career, health, and more. Because remember this allows someone to feel they "belong." Even if the little voice speaks, it is quickly squashed. But this can go on only for as long as you decide—until you decide this belief system does not serve you; until you decide that it doesn't make sense; until you decide that you get to decide what is best for you, not someone else.

Power is an interesting concept. When we look back on history, we see powerful systems that ruled for a long time until enough people started to question the narrative and they crumbled. Take a look at the crumbling of the Roman Empire, or any other civilization for that matter. Religion was definitely a form of power that did and does create wars. All because of differing beliefs.

What does this mean for you? Are you at the mercy of what is going on around you? Do you live in fear because that is the messaging being blasted all over? Do you live from a place of what if? *What if this happens, what if I get sick, what if I spread a sickness, what if I can't travel, what if I fail, what happens if they don't like me* . . . or do you live from a place of choice—to go inward, to take care of your own health and well-being, to focus on the good that is within your life, to be the light and change that you and your community need, to spread light, love, and joy, especially through trying times? Because where you focus your energy is where you will see the most growth and expansion.

I believe that when the noise gets really loud, that is when you need to get really quiet. It is only in the stillness that we can actually find our peace, our truth, our inner voice. We are intelligent, divine beings, but only if we remember we are. Only if we choose to live our lives from the belief system that we are one, we are united, we are love, we are divine. There is no room for fear, shame, and guilt when we remember who we are. When we remember we are one, we cannot be separate. When we remember we are love, we cannot hate.

How do we get to a place where we are so strong in our sense of self that the storm around us doesn't affect our alignment? We practice it every day. Our life's journey will always give us a playing field to practice what we need to learn. We can rise above it and understand that we are always powerful, no matter what is happening around us. We can speak love and not hate; we can be united, not divided.

And it is okay if we don't always agree. We can be on this path and be different. That is the whole point. You get to be you, and I get to be me. If you find yourself trying to convince someone of something you believe in, then stop and ask yourself: Why do they need to believe what I do? Will that make me feel more secure in myself?

We need to give ourselves permission to have different beliefs than our neighbors, our friends, and our families. We need to allow us as humans to live out our lives and follow our paths. That is freedom. If our intentions are not to harm others, then we need to have more compassion and forgiveness for each other. We need to hold more space for each other.

We also need to give ourselves permission to change our beliefs or upgrade them when they do not serve us. That is EVOLUTION.

When you live an empowered life, you not only take full responsibility for your actions, but you also are brave enough to change something because you realize you are ready to let it go. You realize it does not serve your highest or best interest.

For years, I had to work on changing my belief system around living in fear. Years ago, I was always worried about the "what ifs." I held the belief that something bad was going to happen. So, I worried all the time. It made me miserable, and it created a lot of anxiety in my life and relationships. When you are in worry or fear, it is impossible to live in the present. It is impossible to live a conscious life. It doesn't mean not being aware or not being prepared, it means not allowing things that haven't even happened yet to steal your joy, your inner peace. That may sound clichéd, but you cannot be happy if you are worried. You cannot enjoy the riches of life when you aren't present. The here and now gives you magic, and those who live in the moment are the blessed ones who get to witness the miracles and wonder every day, just like through the eyes of curious kids who play and live in awe and wonder.

As adults, you get to do this too, should you choose, but only if you choose to live now. Let go of beliefs that don't serve you and be willing to love yourself deeply enough to allow love, peace, and happiness in your life. You are always in control of it. When the world feels like it is crumbling, you are still in control of choosing to live in the moment.

That is a freedom you have as a human, and no matter what, you cannot have that right or choice taken away from you.

Find the stillness when it gets loud. That is what will bring you home.

So, get curious and find out what's on the other side of a belief system that's not serving you, period. If a belief system is serving you, that's great. As a human, your birthright is to get curious. Your birthright is to have whatever beliefs that serve you, but it is also your birthright to change those beliefs should they not serve you in the highest and best way for this life. Because at the end of the day, if we're experiencing more stress than laughter, if we're experiencing more judgment than unity, if we're experiencing more anger than love, it's time to get curious with our beliefs that hold us to that. And maybe it's time to get curious enough to upgrade those beliefs, for a different reality that might serve us, so that our spiritual and human sides can live in harmony, which truly is heaven on earth, should we choose.

So, what are you doing today that serves you?
What belief system are you listening to that dictates a reality that doesn't make sense anymore?

It is important to bring awareness to what you may want to change.

Think of the top three governing beliefs that you're living by in this moment that you would like to get curious about . . .

Where did they come from?

When did you adopt this belief system? Make a timeline so

you can remember when you first started believing it.

Why did you start believing this belief?

What did you believe about the world around you to imprint this belief?

Now, think about the opposite of that belief. How does that feel in your body?

If it's too difficult for you to adopt that belief, then maybe you need to tailor it back to find somewhere in the middle. Write down the belief in an alternate way that's maybe closer to the belief system you're in now. No one else gets to tell you what to do, say, think, or believe—only you do based on how you feel. That's the beauty of being human. We get to change something if we don't like it, but we do have to give ourselves permission to do so.

So many of our belief systems are centered on the idea that we don't actually get to change. That in itself is a flawed belief system.

So, if there is something that is not serving you, an upgraded belief is:

I get to change this narrative!

I get to change this dialogue!

I get to change my behaviors and actions, and I get to change my outcome if I don't like the current reality I am experiencing!

1. Write down the top belief that has been dictating your life that you want to upgrade.
2. Write down this belief in a different way, a more liberating way. It might mean the exact opposite of what you have been telling yourself.
3. Repeat this new belief as a daily mantra. Sit in silence while repeating this new mantra.
4. Notice how that makes you feel.

This is one of the most empowering things you can do for yourself to start positive change.

We are going to dive into belief systems in more detail in Section 2 of the book. This topic is so important, as it dictates so much of our reality, so give yourself some time to digest now and begin the journey of change by looking at your beliefs.

Beliefs are powerful things, and it's empowering when you realize that you get to control them. You get to change those beliefs, should you be courageous enough to look at where they came from—who decided that belief system needed to be true for you. So, what's an alternative belief system that brings you in alignment with who you really are—that higher intelligence, that all-knowing self?

This will allow you to be in alignment with happiness.

ME FIRST **means giving yourself the freedom to choose your thoughts, words, actions, and beliefs. It means having the courage to be curious about them and where they stem from and to release the ones that no longer serve you or help you live a life built on the foundation of love, kindness, and inner peace.**

CHAPTER 13

POWER OF CHOICE

Life is a matter of choices, and every choice you make makes you.
–John C. Maxwell Source: Talent is Never Enough Workbook

We are shifting on our planet. Our consciousness is shifting because it has to. There are so many things that have been unearthed for many people. If you were living a life you didn't like, you, like many others, may have made the choice to change careers, to change relationships, to change your outlook or what you prioritize.

Sometimes when things get tough, we look at our choices in life and decide to make different ones, ones that will ultimately bring us more happiness, more wholeness, more fulfillment.

What makes us human, and a topic that should not be debated, is our freedom and right to make our own choices. Our choices are what make us unique. They are what determine our path, what create our unique destiny.

Each choice has consequences, yes, but they should never be used as a threat or a fear tactic. Instead, they should be relayed in a way that creates awareness and an opening of minds around the choices people make.

Whenever we see threats, coercion, or force around choices, we should question it as it never comes from light source. As humans, we have a right always to weigh out the facts, do our own research, and come to the choice that we feel is correct.

Fear is the ultimate form of control.

Whenever you make a decision out of fear, it takes you further out of your alignment and truth.

Why have we created so much divide? Well, the first thing that comes to mind is fear. Fear is the ultimate form of control. Read your history books and look at how all the ruthless leaders and times of our past survived. They survived by ruling from a place of fear.

So, how do we move from fear to peace?

I used to always make choices out of fear. The accumulation

of these choices created a life that I did not want and was ultimately miserable in. When I look back now, I can't blame anyone because we are ultimately fully responsible for our own choices. Hence, the word choice.

However, when we make choices out of fear, we are out of alignment. We move further away from our authentic self. In fear, we work from a place of lower energies and a lower vibration. When we make choices from a lower vibration, we attract from a lower vibration. We are still creating every day but from lower frequencies. These lower frequencies create more fear and anxiety, which can perpetuate the cycle until it becomes so drastic or severe that we can't take it anymore. We get so fed up that we are ready to break the fear-induced cycle of choice.

This happened to me when I realized most of my choices were made from fear. Fear of judgment, fear of what others were going to say, fear of not being accepted, and ultimately, the fear of being rejected.

As I mentioned in Chapter 11, we have three basic human needs:

1. Love
2. Safety
3. Belonging

Think about a time in your life when you have made choices out of the place of fear of "what if" or fear of not being safe or fear of not belonging with the masses.

These three human needs are so powerful that when fear is applied, it can create a lot of control.

To live in a more empowered state, a more whole state, we need to realize that we are the only ones in control of how we feel and think. We have governance over our own emotions and our own bodies and ultimately, our own choices. So, whatever you choose, remember it is your right to choose it. And if you feel you are coercing or trying to convince someone else to choose what you choose, ask yourself why.

When we make decisions for ourselves out of a place of love, not fear, then we should be able to stand in our truth and own it and not force it on anybody else. Choice is a human right; it is a birthright we all have. When there is force for any choice, then it is your right to question the motive as to where it is coming from and then ultimately quiet the noise and get to a place of inquiry to find your truth. This does not mean there is no room for critical debate; in fact, debate is needed, as it is what makes the world go round. We should not try to squash or censor alternative opinions but rather get curious and look at both sides, as it creates balance; it allows you to make choices from an informed place that is right for you.

DROWN OUT THE NOISE

When we turn on the TV, we are bombarded with messages; when we look at social media, we are bombarded with messages. We are literally bombarded with so much data and noise that it can feel overwhelming. We lose our minds to the noise.

The only way to get from fear to clear is in stillness.

The problem is that we are so used to noise that stillness feels foreign. For many of us, we are used to living the go, go, go lifestyle until we exhaust ourselves to sleep and then wake up to repeat the loop again, day after day. We create a vicious cycle with the inundation of noise in our heads. We literally lose who we are. We get lost.

There is a common saying that you must think for yourself in order to find yourself.

When we practice stillness, we get clarity of self. It will be uncomfortable at first. It will feel hard at first. But once you practice being in stillness, you will begin to crave it and long for more of it because you realize that the peace you feel, the more whole you become, which is what you are seeking. And nothing is worth not feeling this way.

I have taught meditation to many people over the years, and many of my students initially say to me, "I try to meditate, but I cannot. My mind will not stop and then I feel like I am doing it just to say I did. Then I get frustrated and give up, so now I only do it once in a blue moon."

Sound familiar?

It does to me because that was my story too.

I remember in my twenties going to my first mediation workshop. I actually thought it was like a form of torture. We sat for forty-five minutes on a mat. It felt like hours. Every bone in my body ached, and parts of my body hurt that I didn't even know I had. The more I tried to still my mind, the faster it would race. I kept saying to myself, *When is this going to end?* Needless to say, it took me a while to even try meditating after that. But with time and practice, like anything, things began to shift.

I explain to my students that practicing meditation and stillness is like building muscle. When you want to build your biceps, you repeat the action of lifting weights. It doesn't happen in one session. It takes patience, persistence, and repetition, and it is the same with our minds. When we want to practice quieting our minds, we need patience, persistence, and repetition. And the busier we have been in our lives, the more we have distracted ourselves from the quiet, the harder it might feel. But it is possible and necessary for our inner peace and truth.

When I learned to quiet the noise of other people's opinions, when I learned to quiet the noise of others' judgment, and when I learned to quiet the noise of fear, I could truly start living in my own truth. That is when I could make choices from a place of truth. And yes, there were consequences to making choices that were in my authenticity, but the consequences weren't as painful as they might have been if I had chosen to live from a place of fear.

When you find time for stillness and time to connect to your inner intelligence, you will cultivate more confidence in your choices. You will know with certainty that you are choosing what is right for you. When you choose from this place of self-love, you will feel whole. When you feel whole, you won't be insecure about what others choose, even if it is different from your choice. That is the great part of being human: we can accept each other's choices for self. It is only when we don't feel good about our own choices that we feel threatened by the choices other people make.

Use this knowledge as an internal signal to hold yourself accountable. If you feel threatened by someone else, then ask yourself why. Or learn to take time in stillness to tap into the infinite knowledge within. This place will not steer you wrong. This is your true power. When we realize this power, the truth will flow to us; we will never have to convince ourselves to do something, we will just know because it will feel right.

Exercise to create stillness

- Find a comfortable spot in your home or out in nature.
- Have a timer set for five minutes.
- Play soft, relaxing music or just have the quiet.
- Take a deep breath in to start, then exhale to release your stress.
- Focus on your breath for the duration of time.
- When the five minutes gets comfortable, you can add another two minutes.
- Keep doing this routine until you get to twenty minutes with ease.
- Be patient with yourself.
- If you find it easier, use guided meditations to help you relax.

Please visit the Resources section for guided meditation apps.

Tips to help you with a stillness practice:

1. Use breath work to center yourself (add belly breath or box breath here—see Resources).
2. Connect with your senses: What do you taste, what do you smell, what do you hear, what do you feel, what do you see? (This helps to anchor you in the present moment.)

3. Stare at a candle: This activity can be quite mesmerizing and will help to calm the mind because you are focusing on one thing. If the mind begins to wander, just bring the focus back to the candle.
4. Do a walking meditation: This is a great way to be outdoors and let nature help you ground. Soften your gaze as you walk, be quiet, and just allow yourself to notice the environment you are in by engaging with the senses. When the mind wanders, just bring it back to nature and the environment around you as you walk.

Our world needs more love, not fear. Our world needs more acceptance. Our world will always need the freedom of choice because that is ultimately what makes us human. The power of your choice is unique to you. The power of someone else's choice is unique to them. We need to be different; we need to be our own person. That is the point. It is not to be the same, it is to be different so we can grow and learn from each other and connect more deeply based on those differences rather than making those differences tear us apart. Embracing others and their choices will allow you to embrace yourself and your truth in a deeper way.

ME FIRST **means embracing others and their choices, which then allows you to embrace yourself and your truth in a deeper way.** ME FIRST **means tapping into your stillness to deepen your sense of SELF.**

CHAPTER 14

TRUSTING SELF IS THE ONLY WAY

Don't trade your authenticity for approval.
–Anonymous

We turn down our volume all the time out of fear of fitting in, fear of judgment, fear of persecution, fear of falling outside the so-called norm that is a moving target and one that is decided by whom? Who gets to say what the norm is? Who gets the right to judge you for your truth or actions? Why do we so often give away our power?

In my own life, and a common theme I find in my clients' life, is that misery is often created within our life when we turn down the volume on our truth or that inner voice that is always trying to speak to us that is our true compass to life. How dialed into your truth and your voice are you? Do you share freely, or do you hold back?

Let's face it: We live in a world where we don't necessarily feel safe to listen to our truth. We are constantly being bombarded with "do this" or "do that." Our media channels censor information based on whatever agenda is being mandated at the time. Our family and friends are not short of opinions about how we should live our lives, which comes from their own filters, of course. And most importantly, we live in a world now where technology has allowed a complete stranger to make a comment or pass judgment on what we say or do. Hi, social media.

I remember thinking when I was young about how cool it would be to be famous. The money, the fame, the recognition. But then I would also think about how awful it must be because famous people have their private lives dissected and judged by the public. So, that fame comes with a very high price. But now, with social media, we have created platforms for everyone's life to be displayed and judged. Whether you are an influencer, a service provider, a thought leader, a cult brand, or a local business—or even just someone who uses social media to keep in touch with family and friends—you will open yourself up to criticism. Your whole life, your business, is out there for display. Social media has become this intricate web where perfect strangers have the ability and power to make or break your brand and business. Cancel culture has gained so much more power and control over the last few years, especially the last two. Nobody should ever feel pressured to speak out about something if they don't feel comfortable doing so. To the same effect, if you are someone who boldly shares your truth online, don't let others' judgments turn off that volume. Keep going.

In many ways, I think it has become harder and harder for people to really feel liberated and be just themselves, to live their truths completely, and to speak their minds. Take me, for instance. Even though I am a very vocal person, I have held back, bit my tongue, and not spoken my truth, and therefore, as a result, I have sacrificed who I am and was, only to really understand how true misery looks.

HOW DO WE SORT THROUGH THE SHIT AND DRAMA TO TRUST SELF?

It is not an easy job. Unless you have completely unplugged and live in the woods, you are bombarded with messaging and marketing every single day. With constant messaging comes constant influence and persuasion. If we read an article, we may be shocked or horrified, but what is the balancing argument? What is the other side of the story? Do we ever question that? Whatever happened to good old-fashioned debate where people could weigh out the two sides and come to an opinion of their own?

Here is an example you might relate to: A friend tells you they are getting a divorce. You are so sad to hear it but want to know why. So, you ask them. They tell you all the reasons why their marriage isn't working out. You get the full side of their story and chances are you will understand that they had no choice, or you will judge the other person, and you may even think, *How could they?* I am guilty of holding this judgment, and I have also been on the receiving end of it.

I believe this is an innate human flaw or condition. We take information and we form an opinion. We don't necessarily look at the other side or just simply have compassion for the person without having to *blame* someone for the outcome.

For me, one of the ways that I have become aware of my behavior over the years is by understanding that I can be a really good friend to someone; I can lend them an ear and listen. And I also know that it doesn't make me a better friend to blame the person they are mad at or persecute them without a fair trial. It always takes two to tango, and there's always another side or perspective. That is life.

I remember my girlfriend at the time saying, "You are a really loyal friend. It doesn't matter what I say, you never actually agree with me—you just listen and ask what I want to do about it."

As a coach, not only is it my responsibility to hold sacred space for my clients, but I also must hold it for myself, my friends, my family, and anyone else I interact with. Thus, I felt a moment of gratitude for having the ability to do this for my girlfriend, and her comment really made me think. I guess at the time I remember my grandmother always saying to me, "Sweetheart, one of the best rules to live by is to always treat others how you want to be treated yourself."

Today I recognize this as: "What in me needs to be healed as I am being triggered by this person?" My advice might have looked different, but the same concept holds true. What do you want to do about it? You are accountable and responsible for your feelings. How do you want to handle them?

Understand and recognize that the reaction and response is there for a purpose. It always leads you back inward to self, as the emotion it brings up in you is your emotion, your stuff to look at. Our emotions are a gift; they are our guides in life to what feels good and what doesn't.

Leaning into self-love and self-trust often requires us to wade through the murkiness until we let the mud settle and come to pure clarity. And we cannot do this unless we consciously choose to sit in silence, hold space for our own thoughts and emotions, and witness them the same way we would for a friend or loved one. And as each emotion and realization surfaces, it requires us to have the courage to ask ourselves, *What needs to be healed? What needs to shift? What role do I play in this? What am I going to do about it?* and then have the bravery to face the answers that arise and act on them. Don't be afraid of your emotions; don't turn down the volume on them. Instead, use them as your guide. Your emotions are real. They indicate that if something doesn't feel good, then it doesn't feel good for a reason.

ME FIRST **means witnessing the stories that surface within us and holding deep space for ourselves so we can trust our voice and our truth and take responsibility for our choices and our emotions.**

CHAPTER 15

YOU LIVING YOUR TRUTH IS A GIFT

I want you to think about the times in your life when you needed help and a healer or therapist helped you. Now think about a time when you bought a piece of art or cool picture for your home that brings you joy. How about the time when you might have gone on a great vacation to a spot that was magical and created memories for life? Now think about a time when you might have bought your dream car or dream home that you cherish—a car that allows you to travel from place to place and a home where you create your memories. Can you think of clothing or a piece of jewelry you have bought lately that gave you joy? Is there a program you have taken or an online course that might have changed your life? Is there a book you have read that made you cry or inspired you to do better? I am sure you have watched movies in your life that moved you and touched your soul or simply gave you entertainment. Can you think of a musician or music that brings you peace when you need it or lifts your mood or makes you want to dance or maybe that you play to help you relax at night or inspires you during the day?

We are constantly being touched in our life by so many gifts. These gifts come from inspiration of those who have lived their truth.

Think about it:

- If the artist doesn't follow the path to paint, you don't have that painting to look at and admire in your home.
- If the builder doesn't envision the house you live in or the community you are part of, you don't have the place you call home.
- If the filmmaker doesn't follow their dream to write or produce the film, your soul is not touched in the same way.
- If the musician whose songs you love listened to the doubt in their voice rather than the inner inspiration that said: "You are a musician . . . this is what you are meant to do,"

you wouldn't have that music to inspire you, to relax you, or to make you feel like dancing.

And it goes on and on and on.

It is quite remarkable when you think of all the things that have touched your life—they all were birthed from someone's vision, someone else having the courage to live their truth, someone being led through inspiration. It is what makes the world go around. So, the next time you doubt that inner voice that is propelling you in one direction while your mind is sabotaging or doubting it, just remember that not being true to you means someone else is missing out on your inspiration. Someone else doesn't get to benefit from you being you.

I believe this is our biggest mission in life: **To live our authentic truth and to be inspired.**

And the journey is really about becoming—becoming who you really are, being who you are meant to be, and living from a place of inspiration rather than doubt or insecurities: *What if I am not enough? What if they don't like it? What if I fail?*

All the "what ifs" create huge roadblocks.

Instead, ask yourself this: **What if I don't follow my path? What will I lose? What will others lose?**

And when that voice gets louder than the doubt, when you

really are brave to tap into your true power, it will come to you like water flowing in a river. It will pour out of you. It will happen like magic. Whether it is a new job, a new lover, a new home, or a deeper connection to Source. Whatever your heartfelt desire is. You already have it. You just need to believe it and really be willing to let go of all the voices and messages that are holding you back and are stopping you from creating your dream-filled life. Look at what you have already created in your life. You are creating in every moment of every day.

The real magic starts to happen when you turn the volume up on your desires and make a commitment to yourself.

Repeat the following mantras. Better yet, take a screenshot and save it as wallpaper when you need to reaffirm these beliefs for yourself. Write whichever or all these commitments on a piece of paper. Read them every day to help you stay the course, to help you tap into your truth and to help find the inspiration to be wholly you.

"I FOLLOW MY PATH."

"I am authentically me."

"Only I can and will decide what my unique path is."

"I have the courage to really look at what my purpose is and uncover that gem for me."

"Me being me fulfills me to the depths of my soul."

"When I live from an inspired loving place, others around me will be touched and inspired also; it is inevitable. It is my destiny."

"My desires are nudges from Source or my higher self. I trust these nudges are leading me on my path."

"My path to liberation and fulfillment is my truth."

"My truth is the biggest gift I can give to myself, the people in my life, my community, and the world at large."

When life gives us challenges and throws us off our center, we always have our tools to get us back into alignment. Sometimes we just need help and assistance to get back on track with ease.

When we feel off, or when we live from a place of fear, which is the opposite of truth, we can feel it in our body. Sometimes it shows up as a stomachache, or a clenching in the heart, or a nervous energy around us. When this happens, go back to your breath and anchor in your affirmations to get you back to center.

HOW DO I FIND MY CENTER? HOW DO I LIVE MY TRUTH?

Imagine the tallest mountain you can think of. It reaches up to the sky so far that the clouds cover the top. This mountain is huge and vast.

Your truth is on the other side. How do you get there?

The mountain represents the millions and millions of messages that have been fed to you over your life. These messages are from your parents, your siblings, your extended family, the kids in the school yard, your teachers, your government, the media channels or strangers you converse with in the street, and your boss and colleagues at work. We are bombarded with constant messages, some louder than others, but they all form our beliefs. Our beliefs are based on how we internalize and receive these messages.

When my brother was a kid, a girl at school made fun of his nose. Now, I think my brother is a good-looking dude, and I always have. But it didn't matter what I or anyone else said to him. The compliments that he received for his looks didn't matter because when he looked in the mirror, all he saw was a big nose. The message made an imprint, and he believed it to be true. He lived his life looking in the mirror, and rather than seeing beauty, he was haunted by a big nose.

Our family saw a beautiful, chiseled face with a nose that complimented his beauty. But he repeatedly heard the message from the girl in the school yard.

Her words haunted him until one day, in his early twenties, he came home with a bandage on his nose. He hadn't told anyone his plan, but once he had saved enough money, he got a nose job. His decision shocked us all because we couldn't understand why he did it. What did he see that we didn't?

It wasn't until years later during a soulful conversation that I asked him why he got a nose job. I wanted to understand what made him feel that he needed to do it. He told me the story of the girl at school and said from that moment on he had hated his nose. He had been embarrassed and ashamed of it until he got it "fixed."

I share this story because it has acted as a reminder for me of the power of words. Words are one of our most powerful tools, and most of the time, I don't believe we are conscious of the impact they have on others' lives. I can guarantee that the girl who is now a woman could never have understood that her one comment long ago would torment this boy his whole life. In fact, she might have even had a crush on my brother and that was perhaps her way of getting his attention. Who knows? But one thing is for sure, her words left an imprint on him. Our words are powerful—they can brighten up someone's day, change a life, save a life, console, heal, hurt, or harm—the choice is ours.

So, I look at that tall mountain, and it represents all the people, interactions, or messages in life that have formed beliefs and guide many choices. But the real golden nugget that you will find on this mountain that you climb is "to know thyself" better than anyone or anything else in your life—to know and love yourself so deeply that when a mean or derogatory comment comes your way, it can roll off you or not have a devastating impact.

How do we distinguish between the choices we make based on our core values and beliefs and choices we make based on past hurt? In order to cross the mountain and get to our truth, we have to commit to a journey of self-discovery and self-love. We have to commit to love ourselves so deeply that we don't waver or succumb to others' comments and definitions of what is and what is not.

The biggest healing needs to come from what we most tell ourselves. The inner critic is the one that needs to be healed the most in order to cross the mountain.

Our quest for truth is the biggest quest we can embark on in this life. We are faced with decisions every day, some big, some small, some significant, some insignificant. What we experience today is an accumulation of those choices.

The key is "CHOICE IN TRUTH." Your own authenticity is the only thing that really matters. You will always know if you are choosing your truth because it will feel good and right for you. Your feelings are your guide.

I have learned to listen to my body to help find my center. I listen to the clues it gives me when I am not on my path. We have all the tools within us to siphon through the bullshit and make the climb over the mountain. In fact, I believe that as we dig deep into our truth, we can go around the mountain to get to the other side. It doesn't need to be difficult—it only is if we believe it to be. We just need to be ready to listen to our emotions, to our true inner feelings, and have the courage to follow the inner guide. We need to want to connect with our inner core and truth and not be afraid of it but rather find safety and comfort in the only thing that can actually give it to us: our deep connection to self.

So, how do we connect to self more deeply? How do we connect to our center and use it as our guidebook in this life? I was first going to say that this has been my journey for more than thirty years, going back to when I walked away from my marriage when I realized I was not living my truth. But I believe that it has, in fact, been my journey my whole life. I actually believe it is everyone's journey since before the time we are born. We go through events that bring us closer to our truth or self.

For me, the thirst for a deeper connection to self/Source definitely happened at the time of my marriage ending, but the truth is, if all the events before it didn't happen, then maybe I wouldn't have gotten the inspiration to dig deeper; maybe I would have chosen to live asleep for twenty more years or eternity.

When I think of this, it brings me peace—peace in knowing with unshakable certainty that the events that unfold for us are for our greater good, even at a time when we cannot possibly see how this can be true, and especially in times of suffering and pain. But when we reflect, we realize that these events propelled us and gave us courage or gave us enough strength to say, "Enough. I deserve more; I will not tolerate this anymore."

WHAT ARE YOU WILLING TO TOLERATE?

What you are willing to tolerate depends on how deeply you love yourself. When you choose to love yourself on a deeper level, you will not tolerate crap. When we feel insecure or doubt ourselves, we are willing to tolerate more from others. We have a capacity to tolerate more because it is just reaffirming what we actually already believe to be the truth about ourselves.

One of my clients used to be in a verbally abusive relationship. She tolerated it at the time because she did not think any higher of herself. Then she slowly started making more self-loving choices. She started to eat better, dress with more confidence, and work out frequently, and she generally loved herself more. Eventually, the relationship ended because as she loved herself more, she was less willing to tolerate the abuse. Her partner was not willing or ready to shift, however; instead, he still wanted to blame her for all their problems. In this case, the best outcome was for them to part. She chose to heal the part of her that believed she was less, not worthy, not capable, not pretty, and not strong. I now look at her in awe of her transformation. She is strong and independent, and she motivates others to live their best life and build their own confidence. She has done a complete transformation. It is a work in progress, though, as old patterns can show up, but she is quicker to see the truth of those patterns and make the changes more efficiently when they don't serve her. After her marriage ended, she dated or attracted men with some great qualities, but some who were still not loving to self. She was kicking ass in all areas of her life, job, motherhood, career, and health, but she still struggled with love. I remember saying to her once, "Look at all the things you have been able to create and transform in your life. They show how powerful you are. The only thing that is stopping you from creating that in your love life is your belief that you can't have it all. Use the power within you that has created this great life and believe that the same powerful person can attract the right partner who is compatible and complementary to you." She is now in a beautiful, mutually loving relationship. As she works on her love for self every day, the universe supports that love because she has **decided and committed** to not tolerate anything less.

I have learned this in my own life. The more I work on myself and the more patience I have for myself, the more I am able to love and accept others with healthy boundaries. I will not take on other people's drama anymore, but I can hold space for them to vent. There is a difference. I can love others but not go down in flames if they are suffering. This does not mean I love them any less, but it is also not my right or truth to force someone else to work on their wounds or messages that have left an imprint. I can only work on my own. The more I work on upgrading these limiting messages within me, the more I see the drama for what it is and what it isn't. I used to be unable to see it; I would just take it on and let it drag me down. Now I realize I can love you, but you will always get to be you, and I will always get to be me. That is choice; that is being human.

Finding that center has become the most important thing for me in my life. When I work from that place of truth or inspiration, it flows effortlessly. When I work from a place of limitations, memories, or limiting beliefs, it feels hard.

IT SHOULDN'T FEEL HARD

If it feels hard, chances are you are not working from your truth. Your truth is unique to you and your truth means you are in "alignment." The opposite of your truth is a lie. It means out of alignment or off your center.

Truth/Alignment	Lies/Nonalignment:
Love	Fear
Peace	Limitations
Ease	Challenge
Grace	Inferiority
Unlimited Potential	Overwhelm
Beauty	Separation
Growth	Doubt
Bliss	Judgment
Joy	Criticsm
Acceptance	Anger/Resentment
Unity	Shame/Guilt

ALLOW YOUR FEELINGS TO HELP YOU COME BACK TO YOUR CENTER

How does this feel in my body?

I can feel, and so can you, the difference between love and fear. The difference between ease and challenge, judgment and acceptance, separation and unity. We can feel it every time if we take time to pause and let ourselves feel. To make a choice from this place of awareness. When we speak, when we act, how we behave.

What side are we living on?

But we need to slow down. In order to build this awareness, we need to pause in order to reflect on our choices. We do not want to just plow through our day, reacting and acting from a robotic place because that feels more natural. Remember that mountain in front of you of all the messages and beliefs. These have created human robots, and we can only climb or go around if we are willing to pause and take a moment to become more aware of what side we are acting from—lies or truth?

I was driving to work one day with tears streaming down my face. I remember at the time using the twenty-minute drive to pep talk myself to a place where it didn't look like I had been crying. I had to put on a brave face when I walked through the door. I had 300 employees, and I needed to be a role model for them. *If I came in the door crying, what would they say, what would they think?*

When I look back now, I wish I had just walked in the door with tears streaming down my face. I wish I had had the courage to say, "Having a hard moment. As a leader of this organization,

I sometimes need to make choices that are so out of my truth and what I want to do."

And there it was. My pain came from the fact that I was not in my truth, not living my truth. I was living a beautiful life and running a big successful business that was a dream to do. Just not my dream anymore. I found myself stuck: *How can I get out of this gracefully? How can I leave without abandoning my role and responsibilities? How can I be truthful to myself but not selfish?*

The truth is that we are never stuck. We just feel like we are. From the moment I realized my situation was not long term, I wanted out. Things just felt too hard. I didn't have the passion anymore; I didn't have the zest to want to grow or expand, and yet I felt so limited. In a cage. Someone else would have thought it was amazing, but to me, it was stifling. Running a twenty-two-million-dollar business felt stifling. Others might have thought, *Wow, financial security; doesn't that mean freedom?* But to me, it started to feel like prison because I felt trapped.

When I was ready to look at the truth of my situation and be honest with myself, things around me started to unfold. Sequences of events started to unravel that I believe were miraculous. But those miracles couldn't unfold until I was willing to really look deeply at my truth.

We ended up selling our family business a year before the

pandemic hit. Since then, I have founded my dream business, The Positive Change, doing what I love. I feel like I am more in alignment with myself and my purpose than I ever have been. We sold our home and found our dream property where we can be completely self-sustaining, if we choose. We now are more connected with our children. We have made friends who see us and love us for who we are and are in more alignment with us. With radical truth and honesty comes deeper alignment. Anything and anyone who does not fit that will shift and will fall away. Allow that to happen because that is where miracles will unfold! Leave room for miracles in your life as you anchor into your truth. Become the solution and be the light and change you so deeply seek. It's within you because you are love. You are created from love. And love leadership is what will change you inside out, as well as those around you.

Mirror: "I Love You"

This exercise allows you to connect to yourself in a deeper way. It opens the gateway for deep self-love. Warning: It may feel uncomfortable and awkward. You may cry, and that is okay. The more you practice this exercise, the more natural it will feel.

Sit in a quiet, private place in front of a mirror

Stare right into your own eyes

Feel compassion and awe for yourself

Repeat looking into your own eyes: "I love you"

Notice what comes up for you

Try and do this exercise for a minute straight

Love Meditation: Connecting into our inner power, love, and peace.

Use this meditation to bring yourself back to a place of awareness within you as you open your eyes and allow yourself to feel this love and look through the lens of love as you face your day. (See Resources section for link to meditation.)

Namaste.

ME FIRST **means becoming the solution and being the light and change you so deeply seek.**

CHAPTER 16

SOME DAYS YOU NEED POTATO SALAD AND CHOCOLATE

What do we do when we have those days or moments when the intensity of life feels too heavy? When we notice our old patterns playing out and are angry and frustrated with ourselves? When we slip into annoyance like a comfortable old pair of pajamas? It feels safe, it feels familiar, it feels annoying and yet it is like we can't stop ourselves from participating in the role. We hate this character in our movie and yet there she is, popping her head up and taking a stance that is hard to ignore. So, we play the part and feel the familiar emotions that we have worked so hard to squash or upgrade because at the end of the day, we just don't like how it feels and ultimately, we know there is a better way—a way of ease and flow; a way that has less heartache and frustration. So, if deep down we know this, why does this character still exist in our movie?

As I sit here writing this chapter, I am having one of those days where all I feel is annoyed. I am annoyed with my partner, I am annoyed with my kids, I am annoyed with certain people, but what I truly am is annoyed with myself. I am annoyed that I feel angry and frustrated. I am annoyed that I do not feel harmonious with this day or my interactions with my loved ones. In actuality, I am annoyed with the feeling of being annoyed. So, what can you do when you feel like I do?

Consciously, we can recognize the feeling as something within us, not outside us. It requires having the courage to look at it or take a time-out before we "verbal diarrhea" on anyone around us, which will make us hate ourselves even more. For many of us, we feel we have to work really hard in order to feel love instead of anger and frustration. We know love feels better, we know spreading kindness is the conscious way to live, yet we can be mean to the people we love the most.

TAKE WORKING HARD OUT AND LET EASE COME IN

I have learned over the years that everything is hard work if you believe it to be, and the hardest work you will do is within yourself. But what if on those days when you are feeling angry and all you want to do is eat potato salad and chocolate, you do? What if you recognize yourself as being out of alignment and you approach it with a lightness rather than deep self-judgment? What if you indulge in your comfort food, even if it only gives you a moment of satisfaction, and you just give yourself the grace that your body and mind are screaming for?

As energetic beings, we hold a certain energetic frequency. There are moments when this frequency is higher than others. When we feel out of alignment, typically we are feeling the lower vibrational emotions of anger, shame, guilt, or even lack of worthiness. These energetic vibrations are palpable. And for so many of us, we want to blame the world or people or circumstances for these emotions.

Instead, why don't we look at it as a beautiful message from our body that is saying: "Hey, you are not your highest vibe right now; you are in your pain body or working from a place of memory and old patterns. Because I love you, I am giving you the signs. These signs can either help you wake up and find ease and grace or keep fighting this fight and navigating the storm that exists in your head first and then shows up in your outer world."

We can use this signal to help us rather than resist or repress our emotions. When we see a child behave out of control and having a temper tantrum, we usually put them in a time-out. This time-out can be used to remove them from the situation plus give them the quiet time to reflect and get back to their center. It acts like a pattern interruption and often allows them to have great perspective. Ultimately, the child is able to shift their energy and get back to play in the present moment.

As adults, we need the same kind of medicine: a pause, a time for stillness, a time to realign with our center and get back in harmony. In the quiet space, we can do this. In nature, we can usually do this with ease because we harmonize with the energetic waves found in nature, and we resonate with this as our center rather than anger. But it is impossible to find realignment when we are working hard or are busy trying to change. It's like a jeep spinning its wheels in mud. The more you try to change or work hard, the more burnt out and stuck you feel.

The magic and grace come when we put ourselves in a time-out. When we reflect and let be. We don't busy ourselves with doing tasks that we later resent. We just allow ourselves to be.

To take a breath and really exhale. We open the fridge and eat that delicious tangy and creamy potato salad with no guilt but just an understanding that this is what we want at this moment, so be it. We take a bite of that chocolate and let it melt on our tongue and feel the gratitude of this sweet, delicious, divine treat.

Know that you are divine, all the parts of you. The happy, the sad, the joyous, the angry. They all play a role for your growth and evolution. And the less you work so hard to change and the more you allow yourself to be, you will be guided to the things that make you happy. You will be guided from the place of stillness to moments of prolonged peace and happiness, and you will be guided on how to navigate what you need to find your center—your divine nature, your true self.

It is an unrealistic desire to think you will never have those down days or moments. Those emotional tidal waves are messages. Use them as such and let yourself be guided on what you need rather than try to resist or fight. Fighting is hard work. Fighting with yourself is the most unsatisfying work you will experience. Get curious instead; give yourself permission to pause and exhale. You are so powerful. Your emotions are part of that beautiful, powerful being that you are. Love all the parts of you, and remember, it is in the quiet that you can find the fertile soil to nourish the higher vibrations of joy and happiness. In the quiet, it is much harder to sustain anger and frustration. In the quiet, you come home to self, which at the end of the day, is LOVE.

ME FIRST **means taking the time to quiet the chaos within so you can be guided to deeper alignment and ultimately love.**

SECTION 2

LET'S DISCOVER YOUR POWER + SIMPLIFY YOUR LIFE + BIRTH YOUR DESIRE: THE ROAD MAP TO FULFILLING YOUR HEARTFELT DESIRES

THE ROAD MAP

I have always said that I wished I had had the tools as a kid to know how powerful I was. I often fantasize about how life might have been a lot easier. But then I also realized all my ups and downs were exactly what needed to happen on my journey, and that they created a longing for me to dig deep into the relationship with self and really understand who I truly am. Humans are part of divine energy or Source energy (you might call this God) and our innate selves are love. Love is the most powerful energy on the planet. It heals, it attracts more love, and it ultimately dims the dark and sheds light.

I often refer to my midtwenties as my volcano eruption. It was a time in my life when shit really hit the fan. But I look back on that now and realize that while it might have felt heavy and dark, it was really about me discovering who I truly was and that anything I had built around me and my life that was based on a premise of who I thought I should be or what I thought I should do did not work for me anymore. I had a re-birthing in my twenties when I awakened and saw the world through a different lens. I felt love in a completely different way. I felt awe and magic like I had never felt before. So, everything changed for me in almost an instant. For the next twenty-five years, I was ravenous about seeking more truth and understanding more deeply our power as humans and connection to Source energy.

I knew this hunger would not quell once woken. So, my journey began and still continues to this day. That journey is to live a truth-filled life and learn to make choices from a place of love rather than fear.

The next part of this book is intended to give you a simple road map to understanding just how powerful you are and that you can create whatever you dream up in your mind. My ten-year-old son and I talk about manifesting all the time. He is so open to this language and understanding and the magic that this universe provides to us, once we believe it. But it is not just a belief system, it is actually remembering who we are.

This past year, I set an intention to buy an electric car. The truth is that I wanted to have an electric car for years because I believe that is where the future is headed, and I love the idea of never putting gas in my car again. Cars never really motivated me, nor were they a big desire of mine; however, an electric car felt right, and I believed the time was now.

Six months before buying the car, a series of events happened that I call magic based on the clear desires I put into the universe and belief that it was done, that it was already happening. When we pulled up to the Tesla dealership to pick up our car (shopped for and purchased virtually, of course), my son said, "Nice manifesting, Mom." It made me smile. I didn't even know what the word manifest was until I was much older than my son's age. The truth is that we manifest or create every day with our thoughts and feelings and actions. We are super creators. If we can understand just how powerful we are, we can speed up those manifestations and start living the life we intended to live now. Today, at this moment.

So, going back to my journey, I spent twenty-five years studying and applying these basic universal principles to my own life, allowing myself to become a conscious creator. Being a conscious creator means that you are creating with intention. You are creating anyway, right now in this moment. But when you bring a consciousness to your creations, that is when the real magic happens because you get more of what you do want rather than more of what you don't want.

The following chapters are some of the highlights from my online programs that will help you to become a conscious creator. It is a very simplified process so that you can apply these concepts to your own life with ease and grace. I am in awe every day about how it has not only worked in my own life but also with the success of my clients. Nothing gives me greater joy than seeing my clients stretch their goals or desires and then create them into reality in ways that they could not have possibly imagined.

I want the same for you.

Each chapter will have some exercises for you to follow in order to assist you in creating your desires.

We start with intentions or desires. We then turn up the volume on those by exploring why they are important. Next, we master the process of how our two minds (the conscious and subconscious) are constantly creating based on our thoughts and emotions. We then line up our behaviors or our actions to make the good stuff happen. Once we achieve or reach new thresholds of creation, our desires can expand because we can dream bigger. We can dream bigger because our threshold and beliefs are raised. We begin to remember who we are and that we live in an abundant universe, should we allow ourselves to partake.

Toward the end of this section, we go over tools in the tool kit to help keep your vibration high. We look at ways that you can continue to elevate and expand and tap into more love and joy. You must love yourself first so that you can love deeply and feel more with the gifts around you.

This is where it all begins. Once we understand how we "work," we can consciously create and remember that we are only 100 percent responsible for ourselves.

When I look at myself first, then I have the ability to put you first. When I fill my cup, I have more to give to others. When I fulfill my heartfelt desires, I experience joy and raise my vibration, which creates my biggest impact.

CHAPTER 17

UNCOVER YOUR POWER— TAKING 100 PERCENT RESPONSIBILITY

How to live the life you really want:

Over the years, I have had a longing and a thirst to truly understand how exactly we work as humans. I don't mean work like a job, I mean how our inner workings and intelligence allow us to co-create every day with divine purpose.

I always used to think about how lucky an uber successful person was, or I would catch myself saying, "Must be nice!" I would look at couples who seemed really in love with a longing because that is what I wanted. I would feel jealous of what they had.

Is it luck? Is it good fortune? Is it because of the family they were born into?

I used to believe all these things. I used to believe that whatever you had was outside of your actual own power. It was a higher power, God, that granted you your good fortune or your heartache. Many religions teach that one should be fearful of this higher power, that people will be punished if they do not follow a certain set of rules. I think for a long time this belief kept me in check because I was afraid of making a mistake and then being punished.

Over time, however, I realized that this belief system had also contributed to a lot of my anxiety and stress because I never felt in control of my life. I was at the mercy of "what happens to me" and then I would just have to deal.

If you are one of the lucky ones (which is rare), that's great. But even if you are lucky in one area, I thought, you still have fear because everything else is up to chance. It is like living a life where you roll the dice and whatever you get, you get.

Sound familiar?

I believe that most people who live in fear or suffer from anxiety have a similar belief to what mine once was. They live every day anticipating when "the next shoe will drop" or the next terrible thing might happen. It is like we live life trying to dodge bullets that come from unknown directions.

This is so heavy because we give up an innate power that we don't even realize we have. We become slaves to our lives and are at the mercy of luck and whatever comes our way. It means we do not take responsibility for our life, and when we don't do that, it is so easy to judge others, be resentful of others, and to become defeated by life.

I realized years ago that I had lived most of my life from this thought process and always did what I believed to be the right thing. Marry the right guy, get straight As in school, live within the rules that were set out for me. So, why did something not feel right? Why the longing that kept telling me there is more to this life?

This longing was a blessing for me because it led to the last twenty-five years of me researching, reading, questioning, and seeking a deeper understanding of how "we" actually work.

I believe this thirst for more allowed me to come into contact with some really sage and wise enlightened beings over the years who fascinated me. It allowed me to see humans actually defy their own logic and truly show us "superpowers."

I remember one workshop I attended years ago when I was

doing my yoga teacher training. We were at my teacher's home, and there was a small group of about twenty people who gathered to meet a gentleman who was coming to talk to us about "sun gazing." He was a phenomenon because he defied logic in how long he could go without food, all by gazing at the sun. He baffled scientists and doctors because he claimed that through sun gazing, he got all the nutrients he needed. He only drank a little bit of water for months and months on end.

I remember thinking at the time that it was all quite miraculous. But if we think about it, we hear about miracles all the time. There are stories about people healing themselves of chronic and terminal illnesses, stories of people walking away from accidents without a scratch when they should be dead, and then there's the miracle of planting a seed and seeing it turn into nutritious food to eat. This wonder is around us all the time if we open our eyes to see it.

So, the more curious I got, the more I read, and the more I met people from healers to people who turned their lives from despair to bliss. (Please visit Resources for a list of sages and leaders who talk about the power of our bodies and minds.)

I remember doing a workshop with a corporate group where I was talking about a simple topic of creating work-life balance. I talked about how that power is all within us once we decide to create a change or shift something that doesn't work. Once we understand that, there is no excuse except for the ones we make in our heads that create our habits, good or bad. So, in this workshop, I stretched the audience a bit by talking about our all-intelligent side or spirit side, and one of the attendees questioned me by saying he was agnostic and didn't believe in any of what I had been saying.

Agnostic essentially means that you question the existence of a God or the divine or Source energy.

I understand why many would have this view. I remember when I was growing up that I wanted to believe in a higher power, but I couldn't really understand how that was possible until I went on my journey of seeking. Once I did that, I was able to experience those miracles daily because I could see the world through a different lens. I realize I've diverged here a bit, so back to our power.

The one thing I asked the gentleman to think about for a minute and perhaps demystify the word "God" and his disbelief in a higher power was to think about how we were all in that room, right then.

Think about the following facts and try to grasp how powerful you are. As you are sitting here reading these words:

- Your heart knows how to beat approximately 60 to 100 times per minute.

- Your heart pumps oxygen and nutrient-rich blood throughout your body to sustain life. This fist-sized powerhouse beats (expands and contracts) 100,000 times per day, pumping five or six quarts of blood each minute, or about 2,000 gallons per day.
- Your lungs know how to exchange oxygen from the air to CO_2 produced by your cells. This is called breath or respiration.
- Your body roughly turns over or replaces 330 billion cells a day.
- All your organs are communicating and working all the time to keep you alive.

Now, my question to you is, who is telling them how to do that? Are you keeping track of all of it and taking notes and telling your body how to do the miraculous functions it is doing every second of every day to keep you alive?

He looked at me and didn't know how to answer.

So, I went on . . .

Well, a part of you is, and that part of you is your super intelligence, your subconscious mind, your spirit or all-knowing self. But you are not doing it consciously because it is beyond your human scope to do so. So even if you don't truly believe in a higher power, it is undeniable that we are part of a greater intelligence that is beyond the scope of the material world.

And if we can tap into that power that exists every day and understand how we can live in harmony with our super intelligence, our spirit, our higher selves together with our human, conscious selves, we can create magic and flow and a rhythm in life where we feel peace and awe and wonder because we realize we are part of this creation. We get to be accountable for our life because we are creating it every day. We are not at the mercy of anyone or anything else; we have the power to decide what this life is going to be for us.

We are powerful, but we are also complex, and it can be so overwhelming to understand how it all works.

Over the years through all my research, I wanted to break down a simple process on how we actually can create what we want. I have read very scientific-based books to philosophical books in trying to understand how we work. I do not have a PhD, but what I have done is practiced this work. I have used it in my own life and with my clients, and I have seen fascinating results on how we can create our dreams and live a more harmonious life.

I will never claim perfection, as that does not exist (it is a relative term); however, I do claim to have a thirst to evolve every day. To raise my consciousness every day. And every day, you have an opportunity to create the life you want. If there is something you do not like in your life, you can change it. If there is something you are longing for, then you can begin to manifest it into your life by using some simple techniques based on universal laws of attraction. Every day you have an opportunity to practice a new level of mindfulness with every thought and action and word you say right now.

You have a creation cycle that allows you to live the life you mindfully choose.

HOW TO CREATE MY DREAM LIFE AS A CONSCIOUS CREATOR:

Let's look at this simple process so you can start practicing it in your life and see how it works for you.

THE CREATION CYCLE

In order to fully grasp how powerful we are as creators, let's look at the following diagram that gives us a simplified process of the creation cycle. I want to take you through a quick overview first and then go into more detail on some key areas that are really important in understanding how to become conscious creators.

Tapping into Your Creative Power
Be a conscious creator.

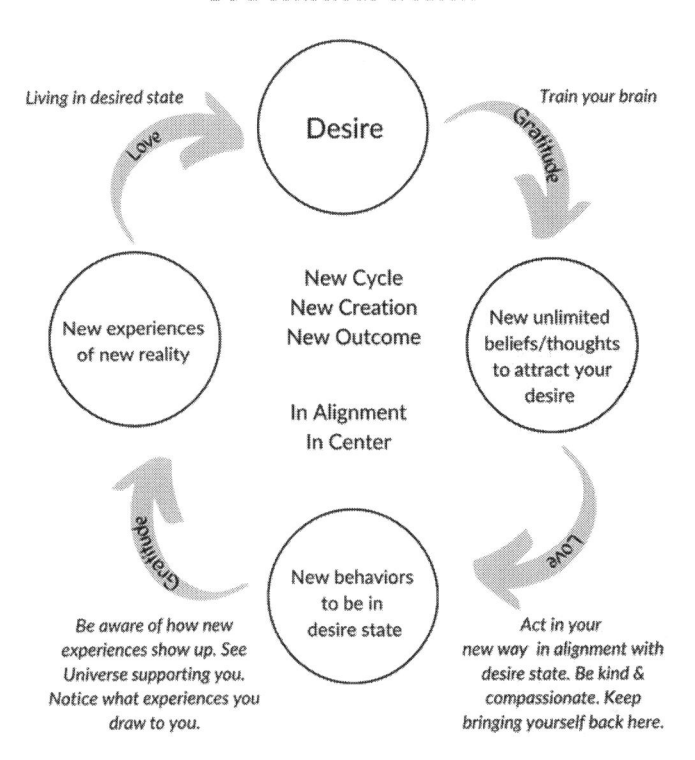

```
                           Desire
      Living in desired state ↑ ↓ Train your brain
              Love              Gratitude

  New experiences                    New unlimited
   of new reality                    beliefs/thoughts
                   New Cycle         to attract your
                   New Creation      desire
                   New Outcome

                   In Alignment
                   In Center

              Gratitude           Love
                          New behaviors
                          to be in
                          desire state

  Be aware of how new              Act in your
  experiences show up. See         new way in alignment with
  Universe supporting you.         desire state. Be kind &
  Notice what experiences you      compassionate. Keep
  draw to you.                     bringing yourself back here.
```

STEP ONE: DESIRE

Desire is the seed to all creation. Desire is our nudge from our higher self. Without desire, we would not have any of the human inventions we indulge in now. Desire is something to be nurtured and not something to ignore. This sounds so simple, but for many people, they get stuck at this first step. They are not clear. I will go into more detail as to how this works as well as provide you with some simple tips on how to get clearer about what you want.

STEP TWO: THOUGHTS ALIGNED WITH YOUR DESIRES

When you can align your thoughts to only be contributing to the fruition of your desires, this is where magic begins to happen. In order to do this, your heart and mind need to be in alignment. Your desire comes from your heart; if your mind is not in alignment or does not truly believe in your desires as a possibility, then you'll have counter thoughts like self-doubt that will stop or impede the flow of creation. When you have thoughts that attract your new desire state, the ride becomes a lot easier. Paying attention to your thoughts is a really good practice to adopt in order to become a conscious creator. I will go over how our thoughts can be our worst enemy and obstacle in creating our desires and how you can actually retrain your brain with a different thought pattern.

STEP THREE: NEW BEHAVIORS OR ACTIONS ALIGNED WITH YOUR DESIRES

There is action that is needed in order to attract your desires, but this can be conscious action that is part of conscious creating. When you create consciously, you will be more attuned with the inner voice or messages that come up for you to take action. Whether it is to make a certain phone call or to read a certain article that might give you inspiration, you will be guided on what you need to do, but action is necessary to create. The difference with this process is that action does not have to equal sacrifice or working like a dog to make something happen or becoming a slave to it where everything is out of balance. Action can be easy and intuitive.

STEP FOUR: NEW EXPERIENCES YOU GET TO HAVE WITH YOUR NEW REALITY

As your desires begin to manifest, you get to have new experiences. These experiences might give you a sense of awe and wonder. Like "I did this" or "I created this." You get a sense of happiness and fulfillment. You begin to realize that you are a conscious creator capable of so much.

STEP FIVE: NEW DESIRES OR REFINING EXISTING ONES—YOU ARE CONSTANTLY CREATING

As your desires start to manifest, you get to experience them and live from that reality. As you do this, I believe what happens is you now increase your threshold on what you think you are capable of doing, and you start to manifest new desires from this place. And the creation cycle continues; it never ends. Every day, moment, thought, action, and reality are all part of our creative self working behind the scenes at all times.

CHARGE YOUR ACTIONS WITH GRATITUDE AND LOVE

Along each step, you charge the actions with an emotion of gratitude. Gratitude acts like a fertilizer. It enhances what you are growing or creating. The more gratitude you have along the way, the more effective the creation cycle is. Any emotion of a higher frequency like love and joy and gratitude will help this process. Joy is so important to remember as you create. If you are not enjoying the process of creation, then something is wrong; something is out of alignment. Conscious creating is embodying these higher energies, as they are truly who you are.

So, this process sounds easy, right? Well, it is easy, but we complicate it as humans. We make things more difficult than they need to be. In order to become a conscious creator, we need to unpack some of the things that hold us back or create obstacles along the way. Once we can understand these behaviors, then we can begin to change them in order to attract what we want rather than what we don't want.

Taking a deeper look at what gets in the way will also help us have a deeper understanding of self and allow us to take more responsibility for our actions and inactions. If we just understood the theory of creation, it would sound nice, but that wouldn't mean you would actually know now to apply it into your own life because your patterns thus far might be doing the exact opposite. This requires not only awareness but also some habit change in order to really get the life you desire. Anyone can tell you something in theory, but how you apply it to everyday life is where the magic happens. And you can only effectively do this if you can understand not only how it works but also why it might not have been working so effectively until now. Basically, what you have done that is holding YOU back. So, let's go deeper into the cycle plus create some action steps to help you really supercharge your creative energy.

It all begins with a **desire**.

KEY TAKEAWAYS

- We are powerful beings, and we create every day with our thoughts, words, and actions.
- We are part of and connected to our higher intelligence, source energy, divine, God (whatever you like to call it), and this higher intelligence is all-knowing and powerful.
- To be a conscious creator, the following steps (the Creation Cycle) are important:
  1. Desire—seeds all creation
  2. Aligned thoughts—connected to your desires
  3. Behaviors/Actions—that align with your desires
  4. New experiences you get to have because you have created from a place of desire
  5. New desires are born—from your elevated threshold
- Love and gratitude help to charge or speed up the creation cycle.

CHAPTER 18

FERTILIZING YOUR DESIRES

If you can dream it, you can do it.
–Walt Disney

The first step to any creation is to get really clear about your desires, your "wants." Your desires are what gives the universe the road map to you getting to your destination or your desired outcome. The clearer your desires, the easier the route becomes to having them fulfilled.

If you compare this to driving or hiking, your desire is the destination spot you have in mind. If you are not clear about that destination spot, you might take the road less traveled, you might have more twists and turns, you might have to travel back in order to go forward, then you might actually change your mind during your destination search because you are really frustrated. So, you put a new destination out to Universe or in your GPS. Now, your energy or gas is being used to travel to this new destination, but you are not too sure if that is really where you want to go, so there are a lot of stops along the way and distractions that come up that take you off course or divert you, and then you might change your mind again because these distractions are just taking too long to get to where you want to go so you become even more unclear, and now you feel not only further from your desire (destination) but also really confused about what you actually want.

Having a desire sounds easy, but for most of us, this is the hardest part. We might have an idea about what we want. Maybe this is what we want, but we aren't sure. So, we give mixed signals out to the universe, which is confusing as your co-creator. And it feels really hard. So, we create goals, then we wonder why it is so hard to reach or attain these goals.

When I work with clients, one of the first things I ask is: "What do you want?" In order to create any transformation in life, desire or wants must clearly be identified. If not, as a coach, I would fail in helping you navigate, and my clients would be frustrated and feel like they are going in circles. Therefore, I always begin by asking, "What do you want?"

It sounds like such an easy question, yet I am always amazed by how hard it is for so many to answer. I often hear my clients ramble about all the things they don't want. This, for some reason, is a lot easier for people to talk about. I believe there are two reasons as to why something so simple has become so hard:

1. We don't give ourselves permission to "want or desire."
2. We don't take the time to nurture this muscle in our brain.

Let's unpack these two points a little further.

WHY DON'T WE GIVE OURSELVES PERMISSION?

I believe there are two reasons why we become blocked here. One of the biggest things that comes up for people or blocks their desire is the awful emotion of GUILT. I have had many clients who feel guilty for asking for more. "I should be grateful; look at what I have; how can I ask for more?" or "Who am I to ask for so much?" When I have asked clients to stretch their goals, it makes them feel so uncomfortable to ask for so much that they feel guilty. Now, I can understand it because guilt is one emotion I have perfected over the years. But when we think of it, it is such a wasted amount of energy that we spend feeling guilty, and it is a very misguided emotion. When we feel guilt around wanting more, we need to understand why. Is it because if we have more that means someone has less? This is a misguided concept that should be explored.

I remember working with one client, and we were talking about money goals specifically. She felt so uncomfortable setting a higher amount of money as her vision. I asked her what the block was. She said, "Who am I to make so much money?"

I said, "Who are you not to?"

"But it doesn't seem fair."

"Ah," I said. "So, you feel guilty?"

"Yes, I do."

I then asked her this next question to help her get over her guilt:

"Does making this amount of money stop or impede anybody else from making the same amount or more?" She said no, so I said, "Exactly. It is not a limited pool of funds. In fact, you reaching your money goals might inspire others to see what is possible instead of holding them back."

This is where guilt is misplaced. It is a misguided emotion that we have adopted for so long. We see it as selfish to want more when others might be suffering. So, we inadvertently punish ourselves or hold back from our true capabilities.

Think of all the times you felt guilty. Now ask yourself why. What was it really about? You will realize you've been holding yourself back mostly not to upset someone else. So, you punish yourself to make others more comfortable about their situation.

The beautiful thing is that when we understand that we can consciously create every day, we realize that so can everyone else. Everyone else has the same opportunity to do so if they want to. They just have to change their mindset around it, and most likely step out of victim mentality and into a conscious creator mentality instead. So, guilt is a false, misguided emotion that only causes one to suffer themselves. Holding yourself back will never make someone else happy. This is a huge illusion.

The second reason we don't give ourselves permission is FEAR.

Fear can literally be debilitating. When we are in fear, we are in flight, fight, or freeze mode. For most people, they freeze. Fear makes them stop in their tracks. Now fear can rear its ugly head when looking at desires because it can be the fear of success or the fear of failure that holds us back from dreaming.

Think about this concept: Are you keeping yourself "safe" by not truly figuring out what you want? If we don't take time to figure out what we want, then we can keep ourselves safe from disappointment. Hence, we limit our desires and keep our dreams smaller.

However, keeping ourselves in the illusion of safety from disappointment leads to a bigger problem in that we never actually reach our potential; we never live out our desires—we keep our dreams smaller. I believe for many, this creates more disharmony than the fear itself. I know for me, that was true. The only way I could liberate myself was by turning up the volume on my desires so it was louder than the volume on my fear.

WE DON'T TAKE TIME TO NURTURE THIS PART OF OUR BRAIN

The second reason we have a hard time figuring out our desires is because we don't give ourselves time to nurture this part of our brain. We are too busy identifying with being busy that we don't slow down to get in touch with the part of us that is longing. We have learned to ignore this inner voice, and instead, we put more importance on our to-do lists for the day. We become hamsters on the wheel, and when we are too busy literally running from task to task, we can't possibly nurture the first part of the creation cycle, which is desire. We are reacting to life rather than creating life. "BUSY" is a word I would often identify with, so I wore it like a badge of honor. Busy is something I see regularly with my clients. They are busy doing this and that. When we stay busy for so long, our "desire muscles" become dormant. We keep putting this part of us on the back burner, over and over again. In fact, we do it so often that most people don't even realize that our desire muscles are something that should be nurtured because they have not given themselves permission to do it. It is now such a foreign thing that it actually becomes uncomfortable when asked the simple question, "What do you want?"

I see this all the time in my own life and with family, friends, and clients.

But what sets the people apart who are living a fulfilled life is that they have given themselves permission to nurture their desires—to spend time reflecting in the quiet to really get to know themselves and their true purpose and fulfillment.

If you can identify with being so "busy," my question to you is whether you are really living. Or are you so distracted by life that you can't possibly enjoy it? And what are you ignoring by filling your day with so many things to do? And when you don't consciously create or make time to tap into your desires, you live from a very reactionary place. This is dissatisfying and can induce a lot of fear because life will inevitably feel out of your control. You forget that you are part of the creative process at all.

So, what do we do because the to-do list is important and needs to get done? Right?

Yes, it does. And as an ambitious person, I know a to-do list all too well. But the problem is that the only time we decompress is when we sleep, and even then, our brains are working for us. How do we balance the doing part with the part of our brain that needs the nourishment of quiet time in order to really get to know ourselves and our wants better? This part of us is starving for affection.

What I have learned in my own life is that when I take the time to nourish my desires and take the time for self-reflection, I am actually more efficient with my to-dos. Self-love is not all about pampering ourselves, which has the stigma of being selfish.

The deeper part of self-love or "me first" is nourishing the part of us that holds the power of creation. We are creative beings that create in all moments—sometimes consciously, and sometimes unconsciously. When we take time to nourish our deepest desires, we can now begin the process of creating consciously. Conscious creation starts with having a clear desire. Then the energy of that desire is planted in our subconscious mind. The clearer the desire, the better root it has in our subconscious mind. Once we align our thoughts, actions, and belief system with this desire, we become a powerhouse. We literally magnetize these creations into reality. Taking time to nurture this every day has now become the most important thing on my "to-do list" because I realize this allows me to be in flow, to create with ease, to be in harmony.

The easiest things I have created in my own life have occurred when I am in full alignment. I had the deepest desire for it to happen, I took inspired action, my thoughts were constantly targeted toward the outcome, and my belief was strong in it happening.

One of my first memories of consciously creating was in high school. I remember attending a new school in grade nine, and I would listen to one of the leaders who was in grade thirteen (we had grade thirteen in my high school days in Canada). She was the sports captain of the school. I would watch her every morning and think, *That is going to be me*. I would mentally rehearse myself in the role. I could see myself standing up in front of the school wearing the leadership jacket and doing the morning sports announcement. For the next four years, I was in full alignment with that happening. I was inspired to be a great team player in all the sports teams I was on. I even remember trying out for grade nine basketball and being crushed that I did not make the team. I went on to play soccer instead that year. I didn't give up. I tried out for the basketball team the next year and made it. I loved playing every sport. I was on a sports team every chance I had. I cheered on my fellow teammates, showed up for practice on time, and loved every minute of it. And every morning, I would see myself in my final year doing the morning announcement as sports captain of the school.

To gain this position, one was first nominated by the teachers and then voted in by the students. I was nervous as shit. But I remember when they announced my name as the winner: at the time, it was the biggest achievement in my life because of its importance to me. Because I desired it so deeply.

I reflect on those days often, and I realize that even at a young age, I intuitively understood how to be a conscious creator. Now, I didn't realize I was doing it at that time, but I would often think back to that manifestation and use it as a touchstone of what was possible when I fertilized my own desires.

I bet you can reflect on a time when you willed something to happen or something you really wanted came true. Think about how you were so sure of what your desire was, then think about your actions, thoughts, and beliefs about making it happen. The more you are in alignment with it, the easier it is to create it into reality.

But the first step is a really clear desire. I gave myself permission at the age of fourteen years old to really want my leadership position. For me, at that age, it was easier because I didn't have the same level of doubt or the self-sabotaging internal dialogue. I might have had some, but it was always squashed by my massively desired outcome instead.

As I aged, life threw its challenges at me, and creation wasn't always that easy, which is what led me to really want to understand "how we work." We are complex beings, and it can be messy. But when we bring a consciousness to our energy and how we spend it every day, we are able to take the full responsibility for our own life and its creations.

So, are you worth it? Are you worth spending time nurturing your desires? I believe you are. Why wouldn't you want to live the richest, most fulfilling life ever? Because you can if you choose. No one can stop you from living this life but you.

I believe you are worth it. I believe this is the whole point to this bumpy, messy life. To live it the best way you can. And remember, you are the only one who can decide what that looks like because those desires are unique to you. So, take some time to deepen the connection with self and really nurture what your desires are.

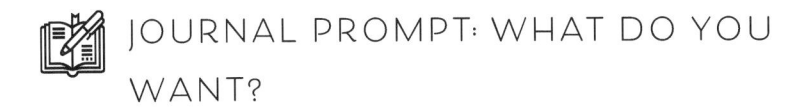

JOURNAL PROMPT: WHAT DO YOU WANT?

Have a journal—a desire journal. I love keeping one so that I can empty out all my desires and then look back through it to see just how much came true over the years.

Write out the top three outcomes you desire in the key areas of life:

1. Health and Wellness
2. Career/Purpose
3. Love/Relationships
4. Connection to higher source or inner peace
5. Wealth/Money

I like to look at my desires often to keep my subconscious brain in that energy. Writing them out with pen to paper actually helps the manifestation process. Then, putting them somewhere where you can see them helps anchor these desires into the subconscious brain.

Focusing in these five key areas of life also helps bring balance into your life. It allows you to elevate the whole you. The point is that when you only focus on one area and don't nurture the other parts, you get out of balance. So, it is okay to focus on one desire at a time, but overall, you want to nurture all the parts of you and set intentions for having it all.

FOCUS ON THE "WHAT" NOT THE "HOW"

One of the biggest things that blocks us from our dreams is that we don't know how they will manifest. We worry about how it is possible, and this worry instantly creates a creative visionary block. When we focus on how something is going to happen, it literally stops the vision or impedes the vision because the vision, want, or desire is overcome by doubt. When we doubt if something is possible, then we not only block the vision itself, but we also send out signals of doubt that make our visions less attainable. This is the law of attraction. If we are doubting, then we attract more of the doubt as well as the impossibility of the outcome rather than the possibility of it happening.

The other issue with focusing on the "how" is that we cannot possibly understand all the ways something can manifest. And if we focus on how it can happen, we literally block other pathways or other ways from allowing this creation to come into existence. At the stage of desire, it is not your job to understand the how. Your job is to be open to the how and to remember that you are co-creating this outcome with your higher intelligence or subconscious brain that knows the how more than your conscious or human side does. When you focus on the "how" instead of the "what," you squash your powerful co-creative ability. Trust needs to come into practice here. If you want something badly enough, then trust that it will happen, even if you have no clue how or when it might not logically make sense.

The biggest key when you are brainstorming your desires is to only focus on what you want. Really turn up the volume on these wants. You might have to start small and build up. That is perfectly okay. Once your desires manifest, you literally expand not only what is possible, but your desires also expand because you have increased the threshold on allowing more good to come into your life.

Growing up, I had many blessings. One of the blessings was that my parents were huge visionaries. They both came from very poor upbringings, and because they immigrated to Canada at very young ages, they both had to build a life for themselves in a foreign country with pennies to their name. When they met and got married, they shared a very strong and united vision—to build success in business and to provide opportunities for their children that they could not have themselves. Their vision was so strong that in their minds, there was no other alternative. Failure was not an option that was entertained.

They would always tell us as kids, "When you want something, put your mind to it." This advice could not have been more true. You need to see it in your mind first; you need to visualize it in your mind, and you need to believe it in your mind before it actualizes. This is how you create.

My parents knew that for them to attain the level of success that they wanted, they had to do it on their own. Thus, they started their own business. My dad started out in the hair industry. He built three hair salons, won all kinds of competitions, and became well known in his industry. However, he had bigger visions. So, my parents changed industries, and over the years, they built successful businesses in the hospitality industry. They did things that seemed impossible. They borrowed money at insanely high interest rates, leveraged everything they had to do it, but never once did they doubt that they would succeed. They just decided to make it happen, and it did.

This kind of visionary influence left an impact on me. I watched them see potential when everyone else thought they were crazy. And in my last family venture, I had the opportunity to work with my dad in creating a winery in a non-wine-making region with no previous wine-making experience. But the vision was so clear that the outcome was decided. It was not without bumps and twists and turns, but we were able to build a spectacular facility, and we won all kinds of international awards for our wine—wine that came from an unknown region, so the awards completely baffled people. I remember when we started, people would say to us, "You will be making a lot of vinegar because what you are trying to do is impossible." And rather than get discouraged, my dad would respond, "Oh yeah, watch us!" Their comments put a fire under him and made him more determined. He was fueled even more when others doubted.

I don't know if my dad's determination comes from years of experience of putting his mind to something and making it work or because he is an extraordinary manifester and visionary or whether it is pure stubbornness. But I do know that everyone can learn from him. Without seeing something in your mind first—with a level of conviction that nothing can sway you—it will not only be harder to create but you will also most likely stop at the first obstacle and give in to doubt.

So, to be a conscious creator, you have to decide in your mind first and not get bogged down by the hows. Just focus on WHAT YOU WANT! And then decide that it is happening.

KEY TAKEAWAYS

- Turn up the volume on your vision; build this muscle and get comfortable with your desire. Give yourself permission to dream.
- Focus on the what and not the how so you don't get blocked.
- Mentally rehearse the vision in your mind; see it happening and feel the emotion of gratitude around it.
- Decide that it has already happened, with a level of conviction that cannot be swayed by doubt.

CHAPTER 19

THE POWER OF YOUR MIND

By now you will understand that you create in all moments. You create your experiences by your desires and your beliefs, but the next step is understanding how it works with your minds.

The things that have come easiest to me in my life have been when I have had a clear vision of what I wanted and when I didn't question that the actual thing or event would transpire. When I didn't question it, my belief was strong. When my belief was strong, any message or thought that didn't vibrate with that belief would not enter my mind, or if it did, I would naturally just shoo it away and replace it with a thought that was more in line with my desire and my belief around that desire transpiring.

I can think of countless times in my life of this happening, when things felt effortless. The desired outcome came with ease. My years of researching and trying to figure it out in my own life made me want to understand more about why it sometimes happens with ease, and sometimes not.

What I have concluded in my own life through my own experiences is that things will happen with flow when I am in full alignment with my desired state. It actually doesn't matter how badly I want something, it is more about being in full alignment with it so that I don't question the outcome. I have faith because I know it to be true in the same way that I know the sun will rise each morning.

But why does it happen this way? How do our minds actually work? I have sought out the answers to these questions for years, as I have had many bumpy roads along the way, and some things that were really important to me did not transpire as easily.

What I realized is that it is not just a matter of positive thinking or wanting something; it is a matter of our internal programming that we have governance over every day. If we want to change the outcome, then we need to look at the programming, the data, we are putting in. Think of it like computer coding. The programming or the coding of the software will dictate the outcome—the actual program created (or life experience for us, in this case).

When we understand that we have two minds, it is easier to understand how we work. We have our conscious mind and our subconscious mind, and when they work in harmony, magic happens. One of my favorite studies has been the teachings of Joseph Murphy. His book, *The Power of the Subconscious Mind*, is excellent at explaining how our minds are working constantly to co-create our realities.

Our subconscious mind is working for us all the time; it is our direct link to our super intelligence. Our subconscious mind knows how to pump our heart, link all the internal workings of our organs, etc. It is super intelligent and super powerful. This is part of us. Now, the key is that our subconscious mind also knows no bias, and this is where wanting something badly will not necessarily get you what you want. Because the subconscious mind doesn't know bias, we can want something but the internal coding or programming that we are telling ourselves contradicts this desire. If you really want to attract more money in your life, but you actually don't think it is possible to get it, your internal programming might sound like this:

I really want to make a hundred thousand dollars this year. I want it so badly. Look how Suzy over there has just said she is making six figures a month. Must be nice for her. How come she is able to do this, and I'm not? But I really want it, and I think I deserve it. Oh, come on, Universe! I am asking you to comply here. Why isn't this happening? Why can't I get any clients? Okay, I am going to write this goal out again and reread it every day, multiple times a day. . . .

This thinking goes on for a couple of days, then you get distracted. Then you forget about reading the goal because you are so desperate to try and make more money. Then you get rejected by a really great prospect. Now you are sitting on the couch eating chips and saying, "What the hell is the point in even trying anymore?"

A couple months go by, and you get another bout of inspiration around your money goals. You start writing these goals out again with a new zest this time. You even meditate on it and repeat it daily. You win a new client. You are excited and feel better. Then you get a disappointment, and you get off your center again; you find yourself comparing your business or life to others that always look happy and make it seem so *effortless*. You start to feel awful again and that feeling of unworthiness creeps back in. *Who do I think I am anyway? Maybe I just need to work harder, pound the pavement more, etc.* And the vicious cycle repeats itself. There is a little momentum forward and then it moves back a few steps again, and so on.

It is so important to understand our relationship with the conscious and subconscious mind when we create. What we program into our subconscious mind will respond to us. Our thoughts literally create our reality. For example, our subconscious mind cannot tell the difference between types of stress. You can have stress over being chased by a lion or stress over a fight with your mom, but stress is stress. And programming is programming. Our subconscious mind wasn't built to decipher between when you are simply doubting yourself and when you actually want something. It does what you say. It is super responsive. I'm sure you can think about a time when your subconscious and conscious mind were in alignment—I'm sure creating felt fun and easy.

Alignment is always possible, but sometimes the programming around what we feel worthy to have or are capable of takes a little longer to encode or to come up with new upgraded codes.

One way to help us understand this is to think of our reality like a garden. Whether it has weeds and flowers depends on how we plant our seeds and what seeds we decide to plant. Essentially, it depends on what we program our gardens to do. Now, I like to equate emotions to water or fertilizer for the garden. When we charge our thoughts with emotions, our flowers or weeds will grow faster.

The emotions of love, joy, and worthiness are all emotions

from your higher self. If you are in alignment with your desires and your minds are in sync, then your inner programming will most likely be charged with these higher emotions. It will be like fertilizer on your creations.

The following image shows how our thoughts are like seeds in our garden and how our emotions fertilize our outcomes.

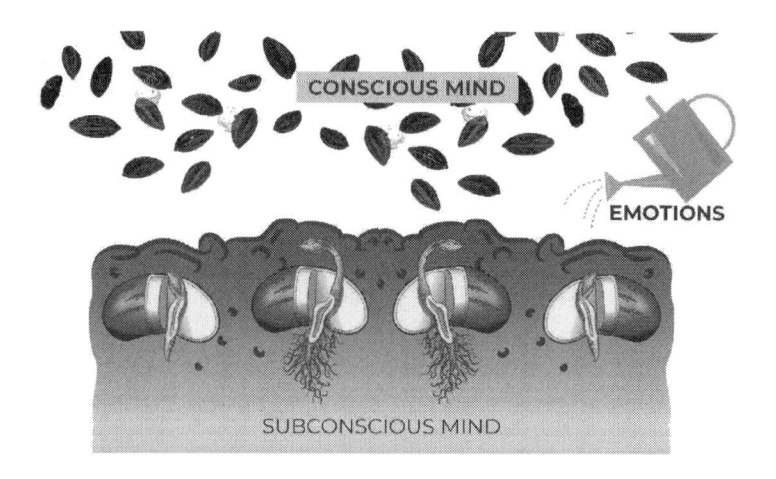

The subconscious mind will take what it is fed. It will not decipher what you really want; it cannot do that. It listens to the conscious mind and believes that you are telling it exactly what you want with your thoughts and emotions.

If you don't like your garden, change your thoughts.

Most of our gardens are filled with flowers *and* weeds. Both serve a purpose, and both are what we have asked for. If we want more flowers, then we need to plant different seeds.

YOUR REALITY

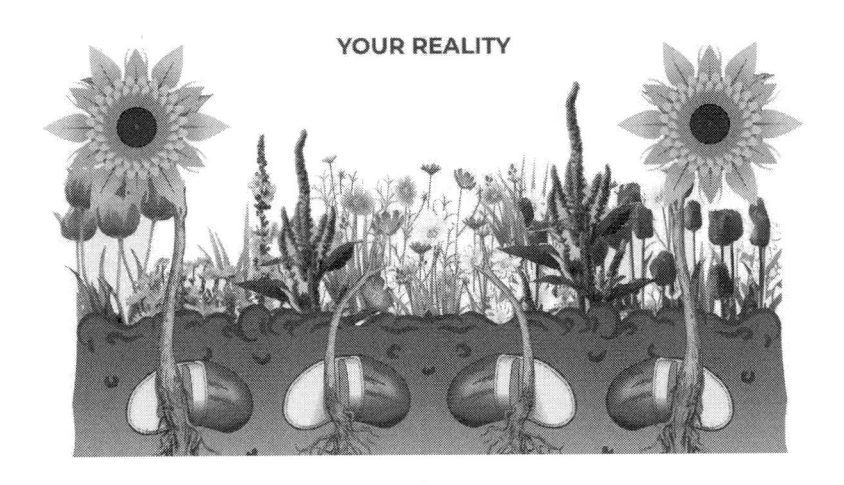

A weed that kept popping up in my life was anger and frustration. It was an easy trigger, especially with my family. I wanted a different reality, but I would too often be triggered with anger. I would look at some of my calm friends and think about how they must have their shit together. They were so peaceful. I knew that to change my trigger, I had to do the inner work; I had to change my coding. Part of my coding around anger was that I did not believe I was heard unless I yelled and got upset. When I got mad, then people would see me, hear me, and take me seriously. This belief and thought gave me a lot of weeds in my garden because I made my loved ones feel shitty and I always felt like crap. Plus, I hated myself a little more afterward.

The new seeds I had to work on planting were:

1. I am loved.
2. I am heard.
3. I am valued.

These were biggies for me, and I knew I had to do that work internally for it to be true. No one from my external world could give it to me. I had to believe it.

I still get triggered from time to time and get mad, but I realize really quickly that I am out of my alignment when I do. I realize that I am not in my center and that I need to look at what old belief is coming up at the time, and it is usually not feeling loved, heard, or valued. I have also learned that when it happens, I can change it around more quickly than I used to, and most times, I can calm my mind first before lashing out. If I lash out, I also know how important it is to apologize, to own my part, and to forgive myself, which is so much more liberating than staying angry at someone else who triggered my insecurities for days.

The most beautiful and empowering part of all of it is that when we can understand the power of our minds and how they work, we can start to plant more seeds that will bloom flowers. We can start to change our reality by loving ourselves a little more and enjoy our colorful gardens of creation. We are all super-intelligent beings; therefore, loving ourselves more is possible for each and every one of us. Some of us may have larger wounds or deeper coding that needs more love and attention in order to reprogram, but it is equally possible. The only thing necessary is that our desire for a different outcome has to be greater than the power of the patterns or programming that have held us back.

JOURNAL PROMPT: PLANTING A NEW GARDEN

What is one outcome you want now?

1. What new programming will you tell your subconscious mind?
2. Write your answers out in detail—all the messages that are in line with you receiving that outcome.
3. Finish by saying: "I trust my co-creative ability and divine timing for this outcome." This will allow you to detach from the timing and fall into faith.

KEY TAKEAWAYS

- Magic happens in our creations when our heart and mind, and our subconscious and conscious minds, are aligned.
- The subconscious mind has no bias; it will not decipher the truth of your internal programming. It will take it literally. Be mindful of what you say and think.
- It is important to understand that while we might want something really badly, it's the messages and beliefs about the want and what our internal dialogue is telling our mind that ultimately create the outcome.

- Our emotions act like fertilizer. When we create from love, we create magic. When we create from fear, we create at a low density. When we have gratitude for what is and what is coming, we add richness to the soil of our garden—our creation.

CHAPTER 20

YOUR WHY

Once you have really turned up the volume on your desires and you can clearly see them like a movie playing out in your mind, it is time to anchor or strengthen these desires. You do this by thinking about your WHY.

Why is this important to me?

What will having this outcome mean for me?

How will it feel?

When you understand why you want something, it will help keep you anchored in your desires. It will help you stay on the trajectory of your creation. When events come up that give you doubt, your why will help you keep focused and secure on your path. Your why is like the roots to the desire. It gives the desire strength and solidarity. It makes your desires less fickle.

Your why will keep you strong and courageous as you create and follow the intuitive steps to manifesting your desires. Your whys become your cheerleading squad. They yell, "You can do it! Remember, this is important to you!"

We all need the whys in our life. Our whys can dig into the emotional charges of why something is even a desire in the first place. We are driven by emotions. Most of our deepest desires will bring in the higher vibrations, such as joy, love, bliss. Our whys connect our desires to these emotional outcomes that we are meant to experience. We are not meant to be angry, mad, or shameful. We are ultimately meant to experience more joy, bliss, and happiness. The lower emotions play an important role in our life because they can propel us to want to feel something different. The desire of an outcome is always to reach a higher state of vibration or experience. That is our innate human drive.

So, when you connect your whys to your desires, it becomes like rocket fuel when self-doubt or patterns of sabotage creep in. Always connect to your why after you have stated your desires.

HOW TO PULL OUT YOUR WHY:

Your why is why you want something so badly.

Ask yourself:

What will having this do for me?

What will having this feel like?

What are the emotions I feel once I have this?

How will my life change once this happens?

JOURNAL PROMPT

Take your top three desires that you are working on consciously creating at this moment. Write them down at the top of a piece of paper. Then underneath, using the aforementioned questions, pull out your why for each outcome.

CREATING A VISUAL ANCHOR

Visual anchors allow us to keep saturating our brain with messages. When we do this repetitively, we can create new neural pathways that become familiar, and to our subconscious brain, this becomes the main language or messaging. The more this messaging becomes imprinted in our subconscious brain, the closer to reality it becomes. When our human side gets in the way with doubt or thoughts that are contrary to our desires, it is also part of creation to our subconscious. So, a visual anchor helps us program the messages that are in alignment with our desires. Thus, the more you read the message(s), the more you anchor in your why. It will charge your emotion, and the creation process becomes easier and more effortless. In other words, a visual anchor helps get you out of your own way. You can also create visual anchors with a vision board. See Resources for instructions.

JOURNAL PROMPT

Recreate this image and put it on a piece of paper where you can easily see it daily. Post it in your office or on your fridge.

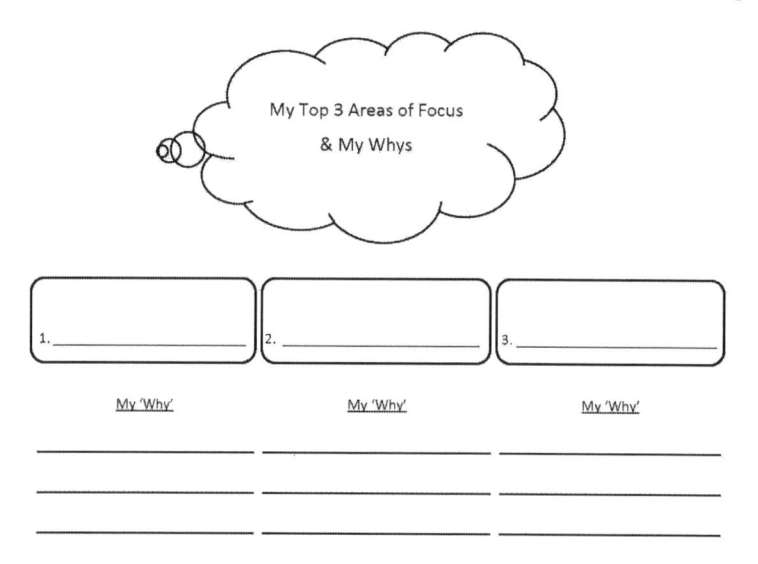

My Top 3 Areas of Focus & My Whys

1. _____ 2. _____ 3. _____

My 'Why' My 'Why' My 'Why'

Many times, the driving force behind your desires is not actually the desire itself but what that desired outcome will do for you, how it will make you feel, and what it means for you on a deeper level. Get curious with yourself, ask those deeper questions, and fill out the chart with whatever outcomes you are prioritizing right now. Anchor your truth by viewing it every day and reminding your brain of this outcome so that it becomes so real it's as if it has already happened.

KEY TAKEAWAYS

- Your whys are like roots that keep you anchored to your truth and on your path.
- Creating a visual anchor will help to program the mind and strengthen the messaging to your brain.
- With every intention, vision, goal, or desire you have, always dig deeper with self and find out why they are important to you. Connect it to how it will make you feel.

CHAPTER 21

WHAT GETS IN YOUR WAY

IDENTIFYING OUR LIMITING BELIEFS

Mantra: "Beliefs propel success."

Two summers ago, my husband and I were trying to teach our kids how to surf behind the boat. My daughter was getting frustrated because she could not figure out how to get up and stay up on the board. My son, who was on the boat, could see her frustration, so he tried to encourage her. He yelled out, "Izzy, believe and achieve!" Now, he is used to me saying all kinds of things like: "Visualize it in your mind first" and "See yourself achieving the outcome you want," but the truth is, you can visualize something all you want, but until you believe it to be true, it will be difficult to achieve. I laughed with my son, as he was so right. Izzy needed to believe she could do it. After that encouragement, she was able to get up, and to this day, she is the best surfer in the family. She makes it look effortless.

For many of the successful people I have interviewed, the common thread for them before they achieved success was their unwavering belief that it could and would happen for them. If doubt crept into their minds, they didn't give it any energy. Their belief in succeeding far outweighed their doubt. I am grateful to my parents because as my siblings and I were growing up, we witnessed them achieving what many would seem impossible. But the constant was if failure is not an option, then you will have to believe you will succeed. I know that it's true in my own life. The accomplishments I have achieved and the goals I have obtained with more ease occurred when I truly believed in them to happen. When things have been harder to obtain, the common thread is going back to beliefs and propelling them.

Belief is an important step in the creation cycle. The first step is the vision, and the second step is believing it to be so.

In order for you to be confident in your beliefs, it is important to unpack the beliefs that have been holding you back in your life first. If there is any goal that you have been trying to attain or reach, and you have been struggling to reach it, it most likely comes down to what you are believing to be true about the outcome or how you are limiting yourself. People often convince themselves that the outcome of the belief is unattainable.

Limiting beliefs are something that we all have. They show up in different ways and in different areas of our lives. For some, they have conquered limiting beliefs around money but maybe they have them about love. For others, love is no problem, but they are limited in what they believe to be true about money and their ability to attract it.

Belief work is some of the most important work we need to do in order to propel ourselves to our highest and greatest desires. It is easy to look at someone else and say they are lucky, to look at what they have or what they have achieved. But luck has nothing to do with it. What we are better to do is to ask what they believe in so as to discover how they created success. Now, there is no doubt that some of us have been born into privilege and opportunity, and that might help to a certain point in some areas; however, it does not equate happiness. True happiness is looking at success in all areas of our life, and when we don't have it, then we have to look at what we are believing about ourselves or the world in order to figure out what is holding us back.

Most people have developed their beliefs from their childhood years. The people in our lives have been our greatest influences on our belief system. Parents, teachers, family members, friends. We need to remember that their belief systems have also been conditioned by their upbringings and the people in their lives who also have their own limitations and judgments.

Thus, for many of us, it has been easy to adopt "limiting beliefs." And for a lot of us, these beliefs have held us hostage in our own lives. The great news, however, is that you can change this programming. You can create a different reality for yourself when you connect to inspiration and source or your true self rather than the limiting programming in your mind. One can see how this gets passed down through generations. The only way to break a cycle of limiting beliefs is when you finally say enough. When you finally decide that you don't like how the story you're telling yourself is making you feel. And when the desire to feel something different becomes bigger than the belief you have adopted, you can create a change. You can literally create a different outcome in your life.

So, how do you start to reprogram your mind with a new belief system? The first step is to become aware of the limiting beliefs that have held you back or don't make you feel good.

I know that one of the biggest limiting beliefs I lived by was that I wasn't a writer. English was never my best subject in school; I always did better in math. The irony of this belief is that while

I may not be the most eloquent writer, I am a writer. I am a published author. I used to always struggle with writing because I told myself I could not write. I was great at public speaking, and I would tell myself that I was more of a speaker than a writer.

Years ago, when my husband and I started our own business together, we realized that the one-on-one consulting would not be enough to bring in the income we needed. We both loved teaching, so we developed a management training course from scratch based on our years of experience in running businesses. In order to do it, we wrote a 200-page manual. We took on the sections of the course we were most comfortable with, and the funny thing is, when I look back at the situation now, I remember that I didn't even question whether writing the manual was something I could do, I just did it. That manual brought in years of revenue for our business and allowed us more financial freedom.

A long time ago, I had a nudge, a strong desire to write a book. I resisted the nudge for many years because it was too scary. However, as time passed, the nudge got stronger and the desire to write a book grew. I put an image of myself as a published author on my vision board. I remember feeling really vulnerable about it because again, I did not consider myself a writer. But I could not ignore the nudge; the desire kept coming. I trusted that this nudge was from Source, or I wouldn't have it. One day, I finally said to myself, "You either start writing your book or take it off your vision board." I was tired of looking at the unfulfilled desire. It almost felt like failure because I wanted to write a book but had made zero headway in doing so. I hadn't even really tried. That day, a sequence of undeniable events unfolded that led me to writing my first coauthored book and then begin my solo. Universe had lined up the opportunity and placed it in my lap, but in order to take the plunge, I had to work on my limiting belief of "I am not a writer." I began to reprogram my brain by writing on a piece of paper: "I am an author." "I am a best-selling author." That sticky note has faded, but it is still on my computer today. I look at it daily. I am reading it as I write this book. I had to reprogram my belief system in order to begin writing. My desire was strong, so I tapped into why this was important to me and then changed my programming. This past year, I have had opportunities arise as I worked on upgrading my belief system that I do not believe would have happened if I hadn't. I have been published in national magazine publications, I am a best-selling author in a book I coauthored, and I continue to write new programs and courses every day. The point is that opportunities keep lining up for me that are in line with my desires, but I had to reprogram the belief system that was holding me back from these achievements. I reminded myself many times that if I could write a manual that brought in years of revenue, then it proves that I can write. I just needed to believe it first. As my son would say, "Believe and achieve."

Let's look at some common limiting beliefs and how we can upgrade them.

Our belief system is what guides us; it is our inner navigation, and when we don't feel good, we need to look at what we are believing to be true about the situation we are in. And when we do feel good, we need to become more aware of what we are believing to be true in that moment so we can tap into more of that higher vibration energy. Our beliefs are directly tied to our emotions. Our emotions are part of who we are, but they also dictate how we are experiencing our life. Our emotions let us know if we are having "the time of our life."

And we should be having the time of our life! So, let's upgrade some beliefs so we can do that now.

I went home to have a quick dinner with my kids before coming back to my office to finish this chapter. Before I left to make dinner, I got a call from someone from whom I was waiting to hear a certain outcome. Unfortunately, the outcome was not what I had hoped. I instantly felt disappointed and felt my energy drain. At home making dinner, I was very aware of my emotions and that I had let the decision disappoint me. The truth is, the decision itself was not what upset me, it was what I was believing to be true of myself as a reflection of the decision. My beliefs instantly went to "you are not valued for what you do." I hate the way this belief makes me feel. It is an old belief pattern that has haunted me for years. Then I had an aha moment while I was cooking dinner. If I could just change my belief around what the outcome meant about me as a person, then the decision would have no weight. It would not matter. If I just trusted and believed that other opportunities or outcomes would come to be that would be more in alignment with my life at this time, then I could trust and believe and let the low vibrating energy go.

It is really that simple. But in order to do this, you need to trust self and source. You need to trust that any outcome, disappointing or not, is exactly what you need at that time. You can either let the outcome propel you by upgrading your belief around it, or you can let it drag you down by falling into a repeat pattern of a belief system that no longer serves you.

I have worked on so many of my belief systems over the years, and it's ironic that a belief pattern that has been encoded so deeply in me had to be triggered exactly as I was writing my chapter on beliefs.

I love the universe. It gives you exactly what you need when you need it. It is a dance, a game, a ride—if you allow yourself to see it that way. And if you do, you can actually sit back and chuckle at what an incredible creator you are to be creating exactly what you need in all moments. You have chances and opportunities to upgrade your beliefs. You will constantly be given these opportunities if you can see them for exactly that: opportunities to upgrade your beliefs—opportunities to wake up and remember who you are and that nothing and no one can throw you off your center unless you allow it or believe less in yourself because of it.

Let's take a look at some common limiting beliefs that arise:

The more you repeat these limiting outcomes or beliefs to yourself in your head, the deeper the programming. The deeper the programming, the deeper the beliefs. The deeper the beliefs, the more you manifest these into reality.

If you want to change your outcome, you have to change your belief around it. So, to begin, become aware of the limiting beliefs you have been repeating to yourself.

The following is a list of examples of common limiting beliefs. Beside the limiting belief is a version of the opposite or the unlimited belief. Highlight which limiting beliefs you identify with the most so you can start reciting the unlimited belief instead. Just bringing an awareness to these beliefs is the first step to change.

LIMITING BELIEF	UNLIMITED BELIEF
I have to sacrifice so much to get ahead.	I create success with flow and ease.
Making money is hard.	I make money with ease.
Life is not easy.	Life is as easy as I make it.
Who do you think you are to be able to want or achieve that?	I am worthy of achieving all my desires.
Good luck—you will never succeed.	I don't need luck; I believe in myself.
We are not rich.	We are lavishly abundant and have all the riches of life.
We cannot afford that.	I am open to receiving money and being able to pay for . . . Thank you, Universe.
They are lucky, we are not.	There are opportunities for everyone.
You are not smart enough to do that.	I am wise and intelligent.
I don't have the qualifications to do this.	I am capable, and what I don't know, I will find out.
I need more experience before I can . . .	My life is my unique experience; it has given me the skills to do this successfully now.

LIMITING BELIEF	UNLIMITED BELIEF
Everything seems easy for her, and everything is difficult for me.	Things can be easy for me too.
Passion fades after a while.	Passion is a priority for me.
You can't have your cake and eat it too.	I can have my cake and enjoy every bite.
Most marriages are unhappy.	My marriage is a priority, and my happiness is a priority in my marriage.
You better work your ass off to succeed.	Believe you will succeed, and you will. Believe you can succeed with balance, and you will.
You can't have it all.	I can fulfill all my desires. I am worthy of having it all.
I don't have the same opportunities.	I am open to new opportunities every day.
I am too old for that.	I am as young as I feel. Age is an illusion.
Everything starts to hurt when you age.	My health is a priority and aging is a gift. I feel great.
I could never make that kind of money.	There are enough riches in the world for everyone, including me. Money is energy, and I love money.

Note the difference of energy in the words on the left side of the page versus the right side. Notice how the difference between them felt in your body. Words are powerful and they carry a vibration to them. The more we work with the unlimited beliefs, the more we reprogram our mind and bring a higher vibration into our bodies.

Now take some time to think of other limiting beliefs that you have been identifying with, then write them down. Pay attention to the voice in your head. Anytime you feel bad or off your center, make a note of what you are telling yourself in that moment. Chances are it's the belief about a situation or how you are interpreting the situation to mean a truth about you.

Dig deep; get to the nugget of what it is. The more you work on it, the bigger the golden nuggets you can bring to light. When we can bring these to light, we become more and more unlimited. Once you have identified these beliefs, write down the opposite of it or the unlimited belief. Repeat these; try them on and see how it feels when you say the unlimited belief. You will need to practice this exercise until your belief in the unlimited belief begins to grow. It is not a matter of just saying the unlimited belief; you must work on believing it to be true.

📓 JOURNAL PROMPT

Create a chart of limiting beliefs and unlimited beliefs. Fill in as many as you can.

TO SUMMARIZE: STEPS TO CREATING A NEW REALITY BY CHANGING YOUR BELIEFS

You have now identified your key limiting beliefs, and now we need to upgrade them. Remember that this is an ongoing process as life goes on and you are a conscious creator. Therefore, more and more unlimiting beliefs will pop up, giving you an opportunity to work on upgrading them.

STEP 1: BE AWARE OF THE LIMITING BELIEF

Writing out your limiting beliefs will help you become more aware of them. Remember that this is a continuous process. The more limiting beliefs you uncover, the freer you will be and the more you will be living in your truth—your unlimited and purely divine self.

STEP 2: CREATE A NEW BELIEF

The exercise allowed you to identify a new belief. Every time a limiting belief pops in your head, replace it with the *unlimited* belief. Remember, this has been years of training that we are unwinding. It will take patience, but it is indeed possible to change the wiring in your brain. Every time you don't complete the limiting thought and instead replace it with the new one, you train your brain. You plant a new seed in the subconscious mind.

STEP 3: WORK ON THE NEW BELIEF—ALLOW IT TO BE BELIEVABLE

In order for the new belief system to work, we need to condition our mind to actually believe the unlimited belief. So, how do we do that? If we've been limiting ourselves for most of our life, how do we now believe the opposite belief to be true?

INCREASING MY BELIEVABILITY IN SELF

It comes down to a fundamental principle, which is what I have been talking about throughout this entire book. It is the principle of truly loving yourself and deepening the relationship you have with yourself. It is understanding who you really are. We can only do this when we choose to deepen the relationship within. We must understand our connection to a higher intelligence and understand our connection to source and what that means. We must understand that we are part of this magnificent creative energy and that we co-create on the planet every single day, and when we actually believe and understand this, we realize how easy it is to create the desires that we want; we realize that it is not a matter of being worthy, it is our job to remember how worthy we actually are. We must remember that we get to experience whatever it is we want.

The best way I can connect with this feeling is through quiet space and in nature. Now, for me, that's a hard thing to do because my programming was the opposite. When I was a kid, and up until my midtwenties, I was always go go go, so the thought of slowing down and connecting inward was actually very uncomfortable for me, and in my mind that felt unproductive; I did not realize that this was the most valuable time I could spend. But as I explained earlier, it is like training a bicep muscle that you want to get stronger. We can train our brain to slow down; we can train our brain to connect with that place inside that is source energy, that is there in all moments. In the quiet space, we are able to feel that it feels like unconditional love; it feels like a sense of peace and comfort; it feels like ultimate joy when we turn off the noise in our head and just allow ourselves to deepen the connection between me and me and you and you. It is the most important relationship we have because when we do it, we get to connect with others on a deeper level, and we get to experience what we truly are and what we truly desire.

When I get off my center, it is because I believe I am "lesser than" or not worthy for some reason. It is when I tend to look at other people and what they have created with envy. When I get back to my center, I remember all that is possible for me. And all that is possible for you should you want it and actually believe in your power that you get to create it, to be it, to live it, and to enjoy it.

JOURNAL PROMPT

How do you connect to your center? Write out at least three things that allow you to feel that inner peace and connection. For some it is nature, music, art, journaling, etc.

SCALING YOUR VISION: ALLOWING YOUR BELIEFS TO CATCH UP TO YOUR VISION

For many of us, we have been limiting ourselves for most of our lives, so we may have to let our beliefs catch up to our visions.

I recommend practicing if there's something you want but you don't believe you can have it. What you need to do is start with smaller steps. Start with something that you can believe. What part of that vision can you believe in now? Bring that into your center, hold it as true, allow it to happen, and allow yourself to be guided by what you need to do in order to make that happen. That's the doing part that we will get into later, but for now, allow yourself to be guided; allow yourself to create in smaller increments until your belief around the creation actually increases. You'll find as you keep creating more and more of that vision that you'll start to realize that you can create *all* of the vision. You just had to do it in steps in order to believe it.

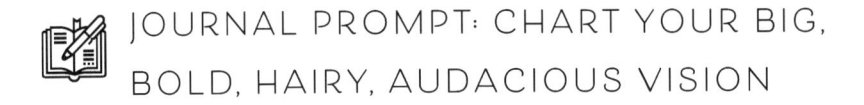

JOURNAL PROMPT: CHART YOUR BIG, BOLD, HAIRY, AUDACIOUS VISION

What big vision do you have?

Rate it from 1 to 5 on how believable it is to achieve within the next three months.

(1 = not believable, 5 = absolutely yes)

Now scale the vision:

What part of the vision or a step toward it would receive a 5 on the scale?

Work with that until you keep chunking it down.

This is what I had to do to become a published author: First, it was writing articles, then it was writing in a coauthor project, and now, I am a solo published author. But my vision was always to be a solo author, so I did smaller visions first to get to the big vision. I had to have my beliefs catch up with my vision.

KEY TAKEAWAYS

- Trust that your visions and nudges are meant for you.
- Carve out quiet time—a CEO day—where you can vision your dreams and desires, marinate in them, and chart their course while allowing the universe to support you.
- Anytime you have beliefs and voices that deter you from your vision, ask yourself if they are true, whether it is your belief or someone else's, then come back to your truth. Your truth is the unlimited version of the belief instead.

CHAPTER 22

MASTERING THE CREATION CYCLE

Now that we have better knowledge about how our creation cycle works by understanding the importance of our desires, the beliefs that propel our thoughts as energy, and the behaviors that follow, we can go back to the creation cycle and take a deeper look.

The issue with so many people is that FEAR holds them back, stops them in their tracks, or impedes their desires from blooming.

Fear represents being out of alignment; we are out of touch with our inner self when we are in fear. Every time you feel fear of "what if," you can use this as a tool or a signal that it is time to go inward. It is time to connect with your center because fear is simply being out of alignment with self.

When we are in fear, we are still creating, it is just that we are creating from a place of fear. Fear takes over desires, and fear drives our thoughts and behaviors. We make choices from these places. When we make choices from these places, we become more and more out of alignment and out of touch with self.

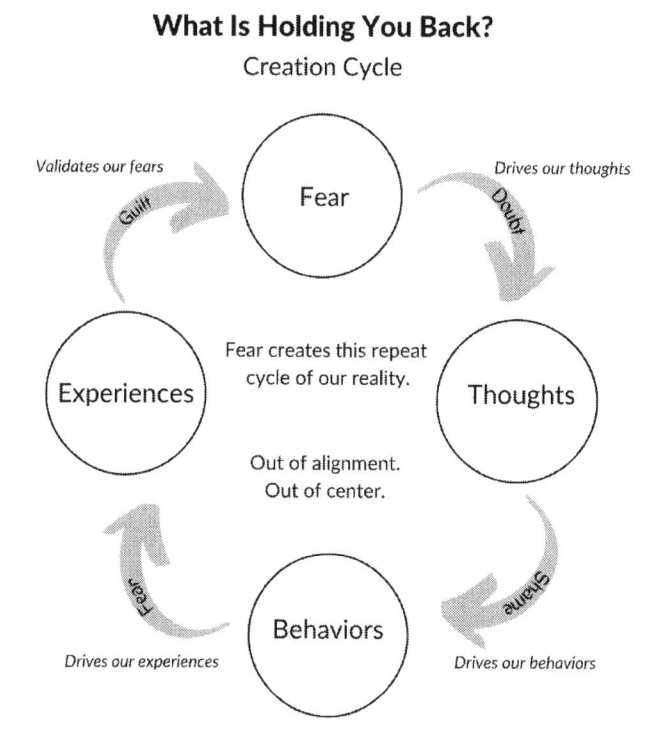

What Is Holding You Back?
Creation Cycle

Validates our fears — Guilt — Fear — *Drives our thoughts* — Doubt — Thoughts — Shame — *Drives our behaviors* — Behaviors — Fear — *Drives our experiences* — Experiences

Fear creates this repeat cycle of our reality.

Out of alignment. Out of center.

Now, if we replace fear with vision, we replace the limiting belief with unlimiting belief, we act from inspiration or love, and we just decided that this is our right. We get this beautiful understanding of how we co-create with the universe every day. We can make our creation cycles work in our favor.

And we charge it with gratitude and love. We feel those higher vibe emotions when we consciously create. Take another look at the image of how to be a conscious creator. This is how we create with intent and get more of what we do want.

Tapping into Your Creative Power
Be a conscious creator.

Living in desired state — Love — **Desire** — Gratitude — *Train your brain*

New Cycle
New Creation
New Outcome

In Alignment
In Center

- New experiences of new reality
- New unlimited beliefs/thoughts to attract your desire
- New behaviors to be in desire state

Be aware of how new experiences show up. See Universe supporting you. Notice what experiences you draw to you.

Act in your new way in alignment with desire state. Be kind & compassionate. Keep bringing yourself back here.

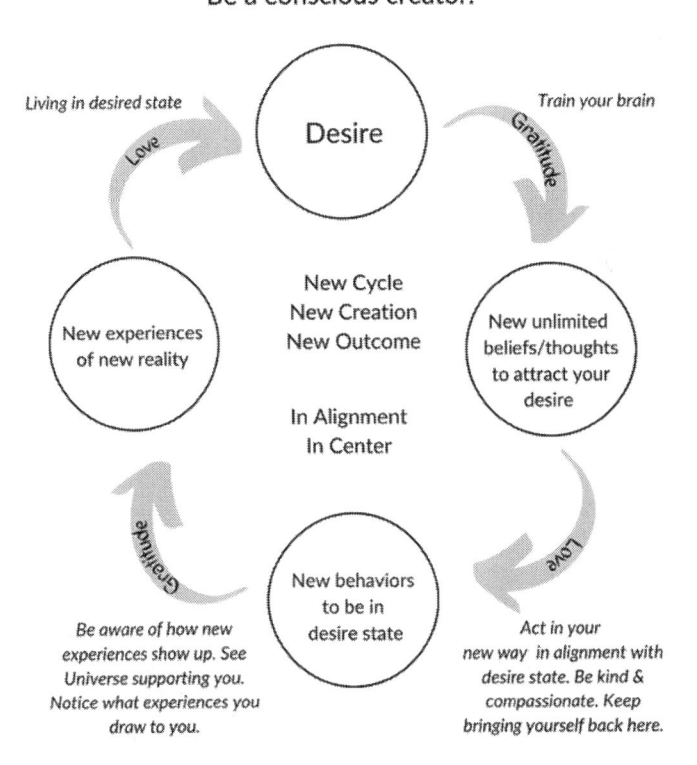

You can become a conscious creator in all areas of your life. Any moment you aren't liking an experience you are having, ask yourself: "What do I want to be experiencing instead?" Get clear on the desire and then go back and upgrade your internal dialogue and beliefs to match that outcome.

For example, I am feeling frustrated and having an argument with my husband. We might be arguing and in a place of fear and anger. We are both being triggered and trying to get our points across, but no one feels heard. This feels awful. But if I want to experience something different and I just expect him to change in that moment, I will be thoroughly disappointed.

So, I ask myself: "What do I want to be experiencing instead?"

I know my answer is love and connection.

My desired state is love, peace, and connection.

But what I am experiencing is anger and frustration.

So, in order to change the outcome, I know I need to match my thoughts and actions with my desired state.

I need to change my internal dialogue from "He is such a jerk and how could he be so mean or do this or that" to "I need to be curious as to what within me needs to shift so I can get to the core of my beliefs around what this means for me." And sometimes, if I do really feel he is being a jerk, I always have the choice to have boundaries and not engage. This is taking responsibility for me. This is the most empowering way I can live. This moves from blame to responsibility for my contribution.

We are the common denominator between our circumstances and the outcomes we desire.

Apply the creative cycle to every area of your life. Try it with intention for thirty days and notice the shifts that take place.

KEY TAKEAWAYS

- We have the power to create deep, aligned change in our life. It starts and ends with us.
- We are conscious creators of our life and can create the outcomes we desire. It requires us to tap into personal power, to share our truth, and to live it.
- If you are pushing to achieve your outcomes, you are doing so from a place of fear. When you are moving in alignment, the outcomes manifest consciously and at a quicker pace. Stop hustling from fear and start aligning with love.

CHAPTER 23

PUTTING "ME" INTO LOVING ACTION

How many times have you watched an inspiring lecture and felt so moved that you decided to make a change in your life as soon as you got home? How many times have you read a book and then thought, *Yes, this is what I need to do, and I am ready*? How many times have you talked to a therapist or coach and left feeling inspired to create your new life?

And then . . .

NOTHING.

Life got in the way.

You wanted to make changes, but your old patterns were too strong to break. Maybe you started to eat healthier for a couple weeks, then fell off the wagon. Perhaps you exercised for one week and then got back into the same old routine, which was not prioritizing yourself.

I have been there. We have all been there at some point in our lives. And then we feel frustrated and angry with ourselves because we couldn't keep up with our new life. We couldn't commit to this new and improved version of ourselves. We feel guilt and shame and are now worse than when we started with his great intention because we are holding those low vibrations in our bodies.

I get asked this all the time: "How do you actually prioritize yourself without your life getting in the way? How do you do this consistently?"

Well, you don't need to do anything. Take that pressure off yourself or it will feel like prioritizing you is another thing on your to-do list. And when it is something on the to-do list, it will feel like a chore, an obligation.

This will never last. This will never have sustained or impactful results. It doesn't matter if you want to lose weight, work out, eat healthfully, meditate, etc. Whatever habit you are trying to create, you will never do it for sustained periods if it feels like work or a chore.

In order for any significant positive change or habit to develop and last, it has to come from love. It can only come from love. It must be part of you rather than something you have to do. It has to be something you want rather than something you feel you should do.

Never say "I have to" or "I should do" something. That just feels like work and obligation. Love is not an obligation. Love happens naturally.

The love I am talking about here is the love for self. When you truly get more in love with yourself, you will not have to put effort into eating well or losing weight. It just happens because it feels better and we want more of that "feel good" feeling. It becomes a part of you because it is an extension of loving yourself rather than something you need to do. You crave it because it feels good. It feels better. You choose it because it is loving toward you, and when you wake up to this self-love or "me first" mentality, it happens naturally. It is effortless because it just is who you are.

Loving self holds vibrations of inspiration, light, love, longevity, peace, joy, and happiness. All these emotions spur from self-love. So, when you are in this place, you are automatically attracted to doing the parts that vibrate with that energy toward self-love. It just is because anything different would feel so foreign or out of alignment with true self.

Now, you should recognize that your habits around positive change and what is loving toward you might be different from what is loving toward me. That is why it is important to know what makes you tick and feel whole. It is important to know what makes you, you.

That is why no one diet or workout routine can work for all. That is why all the promises to lose weight by doing this or be healthier by doing that don't usually last. Each and every one of us has to tap into how it feels for us. What is it that makes you feel good? What is it that feels self-loving to you? When someone else tries to dictate that for you, it will always feel difficult because it is them imposing what works for them on you.

If I make a big pot of vegetable soup, it feels self-loving to my body and to my family. It makes me feel good to make home-cooked meals. I do it from a place of love.

I wake up in the morning and meditate before starting my day. Most nights I meditate before going to bed. I don't do it from a place of "have to"; I do it from a place of "want to" because it makes me feel good—it makes me feel whole and connected to myself.

I lift weights most days a week because I love how it makes me feel. It feels loving to myself, so when I miss it for days, my body and mind crave it. They ask for it. It doesn't feel like dread; instead, I look forward to it.

I like to run once a week outdoors because it makes me feel good. I like the feeling of when I am done best! But I feel like it is loving to me when I do it. I want to do it.

You need to decide what loving you looks like for you. Come from a place of love rather than obligation, and it will feel effortless to develop new habits and a positive lifestyle. Come from a place of love, and you will feel inspired to do what is healthy and loving toward you.

JOURNAL PROMPT

I feel like I am loving myself when I:
 1.
 2.
 3.
 4.
 5.

TRACKING OUR HABITS CAN HELP CREATE CHANGE

Now take those loving habits and put them into a weekly tracker. There is something very satisfying about tracking my self-loving habits. It feels good to visually see how I prioritize myself every day. I am also so amazed at the connection of my mental wellness and my self-care habits I achieved. The brain-body connection of writing down habits helps us to set an intention for the week and to take inspired action.

When I optimize this love for myself, my ideal week looks like:

SELF-CARE HABITS	M	T	W	T	F	S	S
1							
2							
3							
4							
5							

By tracking our self-care habits, we can hold ourselves accountable to self. I also love setting the intention at the beginning of each week by filling in what my self-loving habits will be for that week. It literally primes my brain to take inspired action. Do this practice for some time and just get curious about how it makes you feel. I bet you will notice the difference and you will see for yourself how your week is infused with more joy. You will notice that your capacity to deal with life will increase once you decide to make yourself a priority.

This has had such a profound impact on my life that I created a "Healthy Mind, Body, and Business" Planner. Please see the link in the Resources section for more information.

KEY TAKEAWAYS

- YOU will always be your best investment. Take care of yourself.
- What does being loved mean to you? Give yourself exactly that. Romance yourself, love yourself, nourish yourself the way you desire.
- When you practice loving yourself no matter what, you are able to love all of you—flaws and all. Guilt, shame, fear, and anger have no place there.
- Self-love creates inspired action to develop healthy habits, not obligation. It just becomes an extension of you because it feels good.

CONCLUSION

WHAT IS THE POINT? COMING FULL CIRCLE

Those questions my daughter asked me always pop into my head:

What is the point to all of this? Why are we here? What is it we need to do?

They are big questions, but they have a simple answer. It does not matter what you do or what you achieve. What matters most is you being true to yourself. Are you being authentically you so you can be liberated? So you can be free?

The point is to have fun. To find your joy, to be happy. To live life with the richest experiences possible.

Look at how incredibly we are designed. We are designed with all the senses to experience life to the fullest. Yet these senses can also create great disharmony and misery if we choose.

I can see:

I can look at the world and see incredible magic, wonder, and awe. I can see much beauty. I can be in awe of the magical sunrise that lights the sky with a promise of a new day. I can see the beauty of a farmer's field growing produce. I can look at the colors of the leaves changing and see transformation right in front of my eyes. I can see the wonder in a child's eyes as they learn how to ride a bike. I can see the love of an elderly couple as they hold hands while walking down the street. I can see the amazing gift of a new mom holding her baby with love and awe. I can see the wisdom in an elder's eyes.

I can smell:

We can go through life smelling amazing scents, from flowers to fresh berries to the orange we just squeezed. We can focus on the smell of fresh-cut grass identifying that spring is in the air, and we can be warmed by the smell of a fire in the fall on cooler nights. And smells can bring us back to our childhood: think of the smell of a fresh pie in the oven or sauce simmering on the stove. We can literally be in ecstasy with the aromas around us.

I can feel:

I can feel the grass at my feet and the cool earth below. I can touch the softness of my pillow at night and feel the warmth of my bed with gratitude. I can lovingly touch my partner and feel his response, and I can be touched and allow myself to feel ecstasy. The power of touch can draw so many exquisite experiences once we awaken to them.

I can hear:

I can hear the sound of a child's laughter; it warms my heart and puts a smile on my face. I can hear a crowd cheering as their team wins a game. I can hear the musicians soothe my soul with their magical instruments and an angel's voice. I can hear the birds outside my window and allow their song to relax me. I can be mesmerized by the sound of the ocean waves or listen to the rain on the roof and decompress. There is magic all around us with what we tune into and what we allow to bring us joy through sound.

I can taste:

What an amazing gift we have been given to taste the richness, variety, and wonders in all the food creations on the planet. It is divine to taste a home-cooked meal or dine out and have a chef create a masterpiece of flavors to enjoy. It is glorious to pick a carrot from your garden and crunch and savor the magic of this flavor. It is a wonder to taste clean, fresh water with a squeeze of lemon. Through taste we can experience so much joy and bliss if we allow the flavors in.

YOU ARE AMAZING. You are an incredibly powerful and awe-inspiring human. You are uniquely you with all these amazing gifts. If you slow down enough to just think about the magic that is around you every day in all moments, you will get to experience life to the fullest. You will get to see the riches and beauty in the world.

But with these same senses, we can also see the bad, we can hear disturbing sounds, we can taste awful food, we can feel terrible pain, and we can smell only the shit. Literally. With all our incredible tools, we also have a choice—choice as to what we focus our energy on. It is where we focus our energy that will determine whether we lift or deplete ourselves.

We have been given these wonderful divine bodies to carry us on this journey, and we have the choice to experience life to the fullest. Our experiences are an accumulation of the choices we make every day and the beliefs we have that drive our thoughts. We are powerful creators that are responsible for our good and bad. We are responsible for what we get out of life and how we live it.

You have been given a ticket to the fair. You get to choose how much fun you want to have. You can look through the lens of fear and choose to not enjoy any of the rides or games. Or you can choose to make the most of it—to see the beauty, to taste the sensual pleasures, to feel the joy, to listen to the laughter, and to bring more light into your body and life every day.

We have all the tools for happiness. We have all the tools for joy.

Now it is your choice to use them for enjoying this fair called life.

ME FIRST simply means that you recognize that you are in the driver's seat of your life. That you take responsibility for your own vibration and that you realize when you love yourself enough to live your best life and consciously create and fulfill your desires, you raise your own vibration—and that is truly the biggest impact you can have on the planet.

ACKNOWLEDGMENTS

There are several people in my life that I would like to acknowledge who have been the wind beneath my wings to get me to this point in my life, as well as a huge team of people that I want to give a heartfelt thanks to, as I know this book would not have been possible without them.

I do believe in serendipitous moments in life when it literally feels like angels' wings bring certain things or people to you. When I made the decision to write a book, the thought terrified me and made me feel so vulnerable, even though I knew it was what my heart was telling me to do. Through a serendipitous introduction, I met Sabrina Greer at YGTMedia Co. Sabrina and her team have been instrumental in this process and for that I am grateful. Sabrina, Tania, Christine, Doris, and Michelle, you have definitely been the wind beneath my wings for this book.

I am blessed to come from a big family of four kids. My siblings have been my greatest rocks in my life, but they also humble me when needed (and sometimes not asked for), and they are always there when it has counted the most. Laura, Peter, and JP, I love you endlessly.

Mom and Dad, you have taught me the most in this life. You have proven to me what it means to make a dream a reality, even when it is against the odds. Your message never quit, always runs through my head, and even in the ups and downs and during some of my hardest lessons in this life, I know I have come out the other end a stronger person more in touch with myself, so thank you. Linda, thank you for always being my cheerleader.

My children, Izzy and Noah: You are my biggest inspiration to grow and evolve as a person. I always want to be the best version of myself for you, and when I am not, you show me unconditional love anyway. Jamison, Kourtney, and Taylor, thank you for accepting me with all my quirks and loving me from the beginning when I know it was hard to do. You are three beautiful humans that I am so grateful for in my life.

Rob, we chose each other on this journey and for that I am grateful. There is nothing I feel is impossible when you and I are aligned. We make a great team, and you give me courage and strength when needed.

My team at The Positive Change: Susan, thank you for believing in the work we do and giving me strength and encouragement when needed. Jeanette, you are the best coach one could ask for and after you said to me "you have a book on your heart," I knew that was the message that gave me the strength to take the leap.

My beautiful clients: You believed in me and trusted me and for that I am more grateful than you can imagine. I am constantly learning from you and am consistently in awe of you, and your belief propelled me to write this book.

To my readers, a huge heartfelt thanks for taking this journey with me. Your time to read this book is the biggest gift. I hope this book gives you some peace and hope and knowing that you are capable of whatever your heart desires and that you are always worthy!

RESOURCES AND WORKS CITED

BOOKS

The Four Agreements: A Practical Guide to Personal Freedom by Don Miguel Ruiz, 1997, Amber-Allen

The Big Leap: Conquer Your Hidden Fear and Take Life to the Next Level by Gay Hendricks, 2009, HarperOne

The Power of Your Subconscious Mind by Joseph Murphy, 2007, BN Publishing (rev. ed.)

Talent Is Never Enough Workbook by John C. Maxwell, 2007, Thomas Nelson

WORKS CITED

Tasker, John P. "Amanda Lindhout Recounts Horrors of Captivity at the Sentencing of Her Kidnapper | CBC News." CBCnews. CBC/Radio Canada, March 28, 2018. https://www.cbc.ca/news/politics/lindhout-kidnapping-sentencing-court-1.4596838.

John 8:7 When They Kept on Questioning Him, He Straightened up and Said to Them, 'Let Any One of You Who Is without Sin Be the First to Throw a Stone at Her.": New International Version (NIV) | Download The Bible App Now. Accessed January 11, 2022. https://www.bible.com/bible/111/JHN.8.7.NIV.

"How the Heart Works: How Blood Flows, Parts of the Heart, and More." WebMD. WebMD. Accessed January 12, 2022. https://www.webmd.com/hypertension-high-blood-pressure/hypertension-working-heart.

Fischetti, Mark. "Our Bodies Replace Billions of Cells Every Day." Scientific American. Scientific American, April 1, 2021. https://www.scientificamerican.com/article/our-bodies-replace-billions-of-cells-every-day/.

Genesis 3:19 https://www.biblegateway.com/passage/?search=Genesis%203%3A19&version=NIV, accessed March 16, 2022

FURTHER READING

Dr. Joe Dispenza

Louise Hays

Esther Hicks

Joseph Murphy

John Randolph Price

Eckhart Tolle

David R. Hawkins

GUIDED MEDITATION

Insight Timer

Headspace

Julie Cass https://www.youtube.com/c/juliecass

Love meditation – https://youtu.be/788ydWSWkhU

COURSES

Empowered – https://courses.thepositivechange.com/empowered

Leap to Freedom: *Launch Your Own Biz* – https://courses.thepositivechange.com/leap-to-freedom

ARTICLES AND PRODUCTS

How to create your vision board:

You can also create visual anchors with a vision board. Full instructions to do this are on my website at: www.thepositivechange.com/steps-to-create-your-vision-board/

Weekly Planner: *Healthy Mind Body and Business Planner*

Link to mind, body, business calendar:

https://thepositivechange.com/offerings/

TOOLS TO FIND YOUR CALM

Tapping (p 49), Center for EFT Studies https://onlineeftcertification.com/

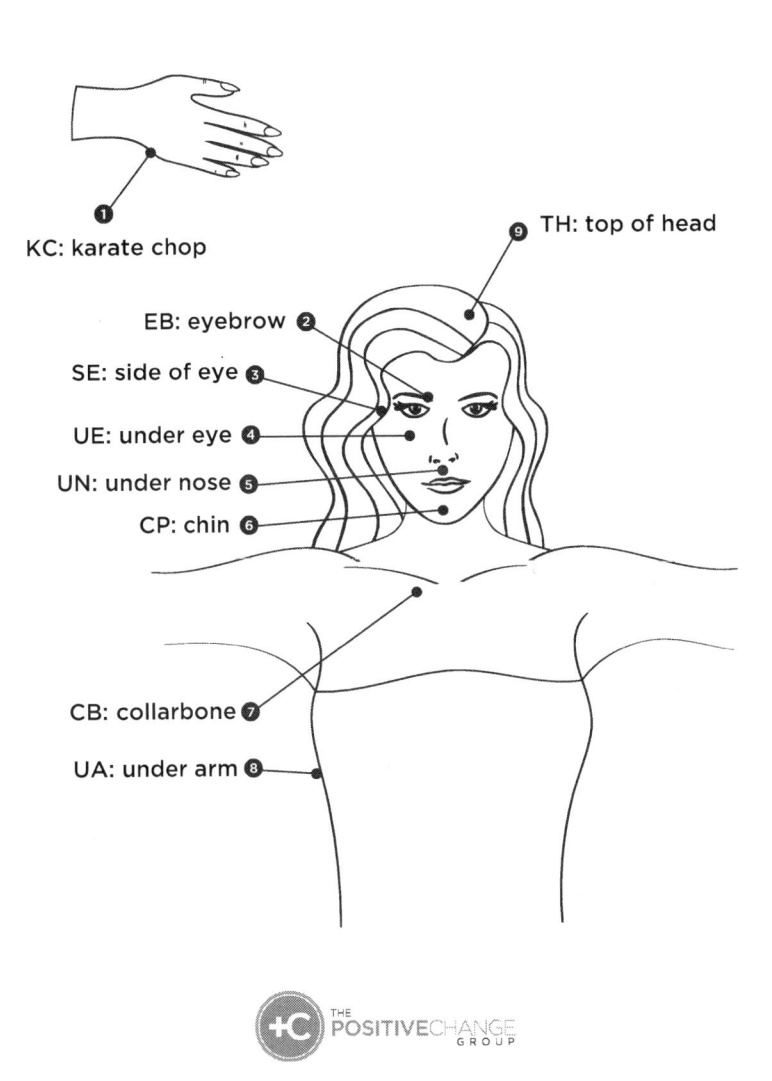

- KC: karate chop ❶
- EB: eyebrow ❷
- SE: side of eye ❸
- UE: under eye ❹
- UN: under nose ❺
- CP: chin ❻
- CB: collarbone ❼
- UA: under arm ❽
- TH: top of head ❾

Belly/Box breath

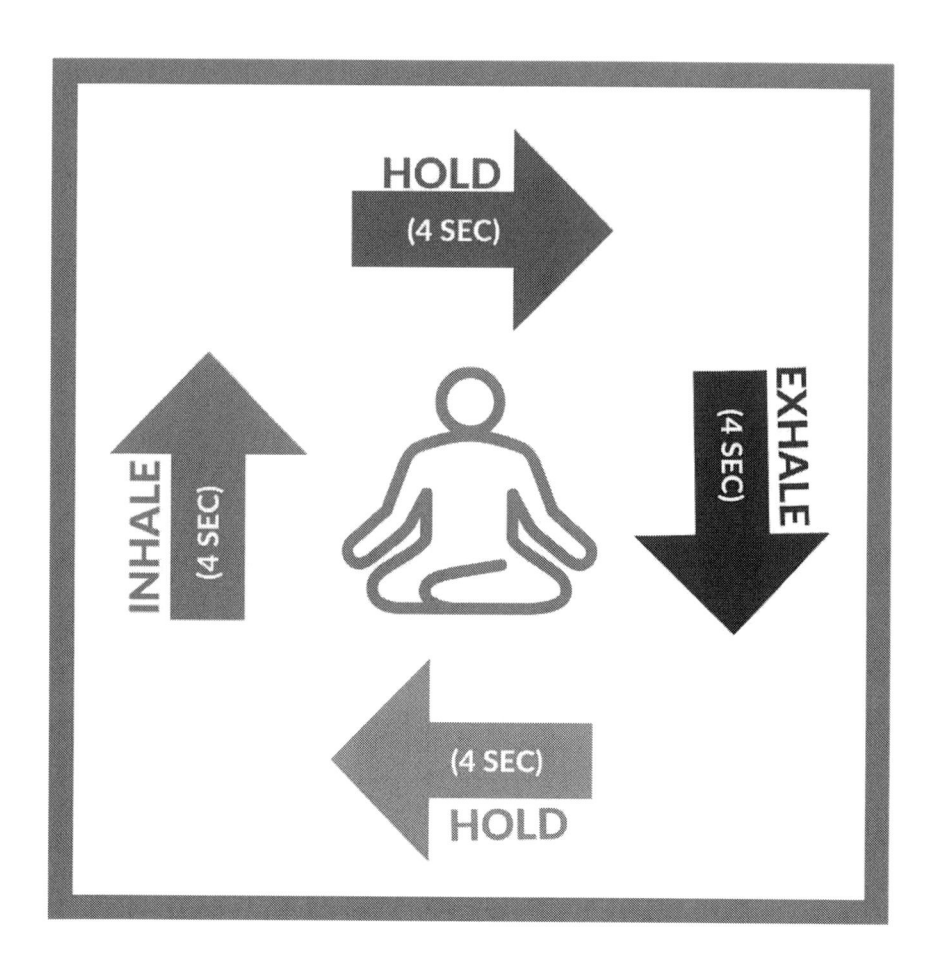

MUSIC VIBES

MUSIC TO SOOTHE THE SOUL

Mike Cohen – Om Shanti Om on Spotify

Larry Ferreira – Binaural Tones for Healing and Relaxation on Apple Music

Emiliano Bruguera – Alpha Waves for Concentration

ARTISTS:

Deva Premal

Krishna Das

Donna De Lory

Ashana

ALBUMS/PLAYLISTS I LOVE TO ZEN OUT TO:

Zen Relaxation by Aroshanti

Yoga & Meditation – Spotify

Indie Yoga Flow – Spotify

Relax & Unwind – Spotify

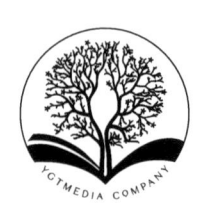

YGTMedia Co. is a blended boutique publishing house for mission-driven humans. We help seasoned and emerging authors "birth their brain babies" through a supportive and collaborative approach. Specializing in narrative nonfiction and adult and children's empowerment books, we believe that words can change the world, and we intend to do so one book at a time.

🌐 ygtmedia.co/publishing
📷 @ygtmedia.company
f @ygtmedia.co